HOW TO (
SUCCESSFULLY WITH

SLEEPING WELL
THE DRUG-FREE WAY

BETH MACEOIN

Wellhouse Publishing Ltd

First published in Great Britain in 2003 by
Wellhouse Publishing Ltd
31 Middle Bourne Lane
Lower Bourne
Farnham
Surrey GU10 3NH

DISCLAIMER

The aim of this book is to provide general information only and
should not be treated as a substitute for the medical advice of
your doctor or any other health care professional. The publisher
and author is not responsible or liable for any diagnosis made by
a reader based on the contents of this book. Always consult your
doctor if you are in any way concerned about your health.

A catalogue record for this book is available from the British Library

ISBN 1 903784 13 1

Printed and bound in Great Britain by
Biddles Ltd., Surrey. www.biddles.co.uk

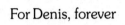

For Denis, forever

Acknowledgements

Working on this book has been made immeasurably more pleasurable by the help and support I have received from the following. Brian Keen at Wellhouse has been as delightfully helpful, positive, and understanding as always, while doctors Anand and Anthea Anand have given up their time to comment perceptively and constructively on the conventional medical advice in the text.

My agent Teresa Chris has done her work behind the scenes with her unerring touch for professionalism and good humour. As always on the domestic front, my husband Denis has been an indispensable source of understanding, practical advice, and emotional support when the going got tough. Lastly, where would I be without access to my very own practical expert on the subject of sleep: my cat Samantha?

About the author

Beth MacEoin trained at the Northern College of Homoeopathic Medicine for four years before setting up her practice and becoming a registered member of the Society of Homoeopaths. Beth has over14 health books to her credit published by Thorsons, Blooms-bury, Carlton and Headway. She also acts as an adviser to journalists on many magazines and newspapers and writes a regular column for Here's Health magazine. She broadcasts on BBC Radio Newcastle and has appeared several times on Tyne Tees television to give advice on general health topics. Beth lives in Newcastle upon Tyne.

Contents

Introduction

Good, restful, sound sleep is one of the most important building blocks of high-quality health. If you have any doubts about this, just ask anyone who suffers from sleep problems how much they would give to have a good night's rest, and you'll have your answer!

Why Are Sleep Problems So Common?

The reasons why so many of us complain of suffering from a less-than-perfect night's rest are likely to have some connection to the fast, stressful pace of life that has become the norm. We need to take positive steps in stress management if we don't want to end up becoming victims of a tense, wound-up state of mind. Sleep problems - including difficulties in switching off, frequent waking and a sense of being unrefreshed on waking - are common symptoms of unmanaged, escalating stress levels.

Additional factors that can contribute to a disturbed night's rest include an over-reliance on caffeine during the day, and alcohol or chemical sedatives to help us unwind at night, plus a tendency to neglect environmental factors that can also play their part in stopping us from winding down. Noisy, poorly-ventilated and uncomfortable bedrooms can make the sleeping hours a challenge rather than a delightful experience of relaxation and renewal!

Bad working habits can also play their part in interfering with sound sleep. These are especially problematic since they are so insidious, creeping up on us slowly until they have reached such an obvious, problematic level that we realise something must be done to rectify the situation. A perfectly common example of this sort of negative working pattern includes the tendency to work later and later into the early hours of the morning. Is any wonder, then, that we find it difficult to switch our minds off when we may be preoccupied with solving work problems until the moment we are getting ready for bed?

Grim as all of these problems sound, there are practical solutions to each one. These positive strategies are to be found in the pages of this book.

When Are We Especially Vulnerable to Broken Sleep?

Even those of us who can normally take a good night's rest for granted when life is going smoothly are likely to have found that we become tetchy, moody and lacking in 'get up and go' if we hit a phase where we are prevented from sleeping well. Common lifestyle factors that can disrupt our slumber can include any of the following: short-term escalation in stress levels, bereavement, nursing a sick family member, the arrival of a baby, or unwise changes in the quality of food and drink that we may rely on in response to an escalation in negative stressors in our lives.

If any of these lifestyle changes occur, it's important to be aware that there are practical measures we can take to get our sleep patterns back on track within the shortest period of time. After all, no one needs the additional stress of feeling powerless in the face of a rapid downturn in the quality of our sleep!

Breaking the negative cycle can best be done by taking simple, positive steps to improve your individual situation. Feeling powerless in the face of seemingly insurmountable problems can often lead to additional emotional, stress-related symptoms such as anxiety and depression. Since both conditions are known to have a negative impact on sleep patterns and sleep quality, it is extremely important to take positive action before the situation is allowed to escalate in this way.

The Individual Response: How and Why Sleep Deprivation Affects Different People in Different Ways

It can be very helpful to understand that there is no uniform pattern to sleep problems, and that a great deal depends on your own individual make-up. The latter is often referred to as your 'constitution' - this term can embrace the main qualities that mark us out as individuals on emotional, mental, and physical levels. For example, constitutional type A may live on his nerves, be highly-motivated and ambitious at work, have a fast metabolism that keeps his weight low, and have a tendency to stress-related health problems such as digestive upsets and a pattern of light, fitful, unrefreshing sleep.

Constitutional type B, on the other hand, may frequently feel lethargic and unmotivated, with a metabolic rate that is equally slow to tick over. Problems that can occur in this type of sluggish constitution may include weight gain, constipation and chronically low energy levels, with ongoing anxiety and lack of confidence as a result of poor motivation. Sleep problems in this sort of constitutional type may take a different pattern, with a persistent feeling of never being able to get enough sleep.

The fact that each individual experiences his or her sleep problems in a way that is unique is of central importance when arguing in favour of the alternative/complementary models of treatment. Unlike conventional medicine, which takes a fairly uniform approach to treating sleep problems (usually a drug-based approach that consists of the short-term use of sedatives), the major systems of alternative medicine described in this book take a rather different perspective.

From an alternative medical viewpoint, effective treatment for a chronic, well-established problem such as poor or interrupted sleep patterns can be established once enough of the patient's individual features and unique circumstances have been identified. In other words, alternative therapists tend to be more interested in the differences that exist between one patient's insomnia and another's than in the common features they share. This is likely to be the case whether you consult a homoeopath, traditional Chinese practitioner, Western medical herbalist or Ayurvedic practitioner (more detailed explanations of the theory and practical application of a selection of alternative and complementary therapies can be found in Chapter Seven).

Chapter One

The Importance of Sleep

It is impossible to work as a homoeopathic practitioner and be unaware of the vitally important role that a balanced sleep pattern plays in ensuring a sense of optimum well-being and good health. Broken sleep or any kind of unrefreshing sleep pattern is almost certainly one of the most obvious precursors of a phase of ill-health. As a result, I have very seldom come across a patient who admits to having had a refreshing night's sleep just prior to or since developing symptoms of ill-health.

However, it is also important to establish at the outset that what is most important here is the *quality* of your sleep, rather than the number of hours spent at rest. In other words, for many patients the problem is not a difficulty in switching off, but more a struggle to get themselves pulled around in the morning. These are the unfortunate patients who feel they just can't get enough hours' sleep, because they never feel refreshed on waking. As a result, even 10 hours or so of slumber, if it is unsatisfactory, can leave them feeling thick-headed and fuzzy, since they feel they have hardly been asleep at all.

As mentioned in the Introduction, we all have individual needs in the sleep department, and each of us probably has an instinctive sense of what we know is the duration and depth of an optimum night's rest for us. Any marked departure from this pattern for a noticeable length of time, and we need to consider using practical strategies in order to get our sleep patterns back on track. We should make this a priority because of the undeniable impact that sleep patterns have on our emotional, mental and physical health.

Although some aspects of sleep remain a mystery, we know that a regular, healthy sleep pattern allows our internal organs a much-needed rest and chance for renewal, while the psychological benefits that come from dreaming appear to be vitally important in allowing us to work through the mental and emotional pressures of our day.

Sleep and Recurrent Infections

Immune-system functioning also appears to be adversely affected by long-term sleep disruption, resulting in poor resistance to infections and a general sense of being run down. Studies have shown that sleep deprivation, even of only one or two days in young, healthy people, can reduce the number of 'killer' cells produced by the immune system to fight off infection. As a result, the longer our sleep problems go on, the greater the chance that we'll be unable to fight off cold and flu viruses effectively.

The healing effect of sleep is something many of us may have experienced at first hand if we've suffered from an acute illness like a heavy cold, flu or a gastric upset as a result of catching a bug or eating something that has become contaminated. It's the most natural thing in the world when we're ill to feel we just want to take to a warm bed and sleep the worst of the symptoms off.

Since we are aware that sleep can have a boosting effect on the immune system, it makes sense that regular, refreshing, sound sleep helps to bolster our resistance to infection and may also play an important role in helping us fight off acute illnesses more decisively and efficiently. And if we do suffer a bout of acute illness, getting proper rest can help shorten its duration, as well as possibly lessening the risk of developing complications.

Sleep and Balanced Mental and Emotional Health

Experiencing the benefits of a regular, sound sleep pattern also has a profound effect on our mental and emotional balance. Lack of sound, refreshing sleep on an ongoing basis can leave us feeling irritable, indecisive and prone to errors in judgement. Anyone who has been up regularly night after night caring for a young baby is likely to be able to speak first hand about the emotional 'short-fuse' that is the almost inevitable knock-on effect during the day. This combination of easily triggered irritability and irrationality tends to build in a cumulative way as we are deprived of increasing hours of sleep.

Poor memory can also be a direct legacy of lack of rest, which can make us feel under ever-increasing pressure. This often has the additional effect of making us feel generally stressed and anxious, which is likely to render us more vulnerable to poor sleep patterns. This can lead to a negative cycle, where feeling emotionally, mentally and physically tense about our sleep problems makes it increasingly unlikely that we are going to switch off effectively at night.

This negative cycle can be further compounded by adopting 'quick-fix' coping mechanisms that seem to work in the short term but only lead to further problems down the line. These can include reaching for caffeine 'shots' during the day in order to give ourselves a temporary boost, and relying on a stiff drink or two and/or sleeping pills at night in order to wind down. You will learn how to say good-bye to these counter-productive strategies in Chapter Five.

Cosmetic Benefits of Sleep

When we sleep well, there are additional benefits in the form of healthy skin tone, brighter eyes and a reduced tendency to develop dark bags and puffiness around the eyes. The anti-ageing effect of a healthy sleep pattern appears to be due to the relationship between the secretion of growth hormone and sound sleep patterns. Not only is optimum secretion of growth hormone absolutely essential in encouraging healthy growth patterns and development in young children, but it plays a significant role for adults, too.

The healthy secretion of growth hormone in adults ensures the proper renewal and repair of body cells. As a result, a wide range of body cells including those that make up our skin, blood and vital organs such as the brain are thought to be renewed faster when we are sleeping soundly than when we are fully conscious and active.

Sleep and Persistent Fatigue

The relationship between a healthy sleep pattern and sustained, optimum levels of energy really speaks for itself. After all, who hasn't experienced the perceptible energy slump that follows a period of lack of sleep?

The complicating factor associated with this sort of fatigue is that it feels so all-encompassing. In other words, this is not just a profound sense of physical tiredness, but it brings with it a profound sense of mental fatigue. The situation may be intensified if we develop the habit of reaching for drinks that are marketed as 'energy-boosting'. Unfortunately, while these give a temporary mental and physical energy 'buzz', there is a high price to be paid if we rely on them in the long run. These products will be discussed in Chapter Five.

The dangers of the deep-seated fatigue that is a consequence of sleep deprivation have been well publicised recently. The number of serious road traffic accidents that can be attributed to the driver having nodded off at the wheel is alarmingly high. It has been estimated by the British Sleep Foundation that drowsy drivers are responsible for an alarming 20 per cent of road traffic accidents. A no less worrying situation exists in the United States, where the National Highway Traffic Safety Administration claims that there are approximately 100,000 car accidents in the US each year caused by sleepy drivers. Of these accidents, approximately 1,500 have fatal consequences.

Tasks that require a sharp level of concentration and co-ordination can also suffer, making working with machinery a hazard if we are sleepy and lacking in mental focus.

These serious risks apart, there is also an equally worrying aspect of long-term fatigue which negatively affects the quality of life that we enjoy on a day-to-day basis. Feeling tired all of the time takes the pleasurable edge and excitement off so many aspects of life. Socialising with friends, planning a meal, going to the cinema, making love or having the enthusiasm to play with young children all require a healthy supply of energy if we are to derive maximum pleasure from these experiences.

And this is before we even consider the impact that flagging levels of vitality can have on our performance at work. Knowing that we feel mentally and physically sluggish and lacking in a healthy competitive drive is something that most of us are likely to find deeply stressful if it goes on for any noticeable length of time. The unpleasant irony is that this sort of stress can make it even more difficult for us to achieve what we need most: a refreshing, unbroken night's sleep.

This problem can emerge as a knock-on effect of persistent fatigue caused by lack of sleep. Many of the migraine sufferers whom I have treated have established that becoming excessively tired through lack of sleep will almost certainly trigger an acute episode of migraine.

Those who do not suffer from full-blown migraines, but are subject more often to tension headaches, have also noticed that sleep loss caused by being under acute professional or domestic stress can result in almost daily tension headaches.

Unfortunately this results in a particularly frustrating vicious circle, where long-term problems with lack of sleep cause a sense of physical and mental anxiety to develop. This, in turn, makes it likely that a great deal of muscular tension builds up in the jaw, face, neck and shoulders. A tendency towards tooth-grinding is an almost certain sign that this is the problem. Once this negative situation is established, blood flow to the head and scalp muscles can be adversely affected, leading to regular problems with tension headaches. This can be aggravated by postural problems, including those brought on by watching television in bed, where there is a natural tendency to prop the head forward while watching the screen. Of course, watching television late at night in bed is also unlikely to encourage us to go off peacefully to sleep, since so many programmes create a sense of stimulation rather than relaxation.

How the Ageing Process Affects the Amount of Sleep We Need

Most of us will be aware that our sleep requirements change, not just according to the demands that are being made of us (for instance, many pregnant women find in the first three months that they feel constantly tired and in need of more sleep), but also according to our age.

Babies, for instance, need to sleep for a sizable proportion of each day, with a gradual emergence of a sleep pattern happening as maturity develops. Interestingly, there is no hard-and-fast pattern to this development, since some babies settle to sleeping through the night within weeks (these, of course, are the ones whose parents consider themselves incredibly lucky!), while others reach toddler-hood still finding it difficult to rest through the night.

The same variables can affect us in youth and middle age, since some of us have constitutions that require a very short period of sleep in order to function to maximum capacity (this can be as short as three or four hours), while others know that they must have a full, unbroken eight hours of good quality rest.

Once we move beyond middle age into what has been termed 'the third age' (in other words, over 60), our sleep requirements are likely to have changed once again. As there is a change in the rhythm of our daily lives as a result of retirement, with more hours of leisure time available to us, we may find that we are able to thrive on a reduced number of hours of sleep at night.

Some over-60s may find, since they are sleeping for fewer hours at night, that they benefit from a short nap during the day when their energy levels are at a low ebb. On the other hand, others may feel that their constitutional profile reacts very badly to a short sleep during the day, leaving them feeling anything but energised or refreshed.

Additional factors that can affect our sleep requirements include hormonal changes, especially in pre-menstrual women who frequently find that their sleep patterns change at ovulation (mid-cycle) or for a night or so before their period arrives. Sleep demands also increase steadily during the period of adolescence, an obvious stage of hormonal development in girls and boys alike.

At the other end of the spectrum, women approaching or going through the menopause can also find that their sleep patterns undergo quite a transformation. Anything from mild to severe insomnia is a common symptom of the menopause. This can be linked to the emergence of night sweats (which clearly don't do a great deal to encourage a sound night's rest!). Even women who do not suffer hot flushes or night sweats can find that they wake frequently during the night, or find it extremely difficult to switch off and get into a sound sleep as a result of menopausal changes..

Having said this, there are some benefits to going through menopause, since studies have revealed that menopausal women tend to get optimum phases of deep sleep per night. In the next chapter we will explore what we mean by deep sleep, the various phases of sleep we go through each night and the benefits they bring.

At-a-Glance Breakdown of Sleep Patterns through Major Phases of Life

Although sleep requirements can vary greatly from one person to another, the following table gives some very rough guidelines to the way our sleep patterns and phases can change as we move through the major transitional benchmarks in life.

Phase of Life Sleep Requirements	
Newborns and children	A young baby can nap for anything up to an astonishing 18 hours a day. As they mature, children spend fewer total hours asleep, but sleep for longer periods at a stretch. By 3 or 4 years of age, a child will spend 3 or 4 hours in REM sleep and approximately 5 hours in light sleep. The portion of REM sleep reduces to an adult proportion of up to 2 hours each night by the time a child reaches the age of 10.
Adolescents	By the teenage years, the need for sleep temporarily increases, although time spent in deep sleep decreases.
Adults	Sleep patterns should reach their cruising levels by age 20 to 30. An average night should include roughly 7 to 8 hours' sleep, which is likely to be made up of approximately 4 hours of light sleep, only 1½ hours of deep sleep, and the remainder REM activity.
Seniors	Around the age of 50, sleep requirements begin to change for men and women alike. Overall time spent asleep will generally decrease over the years, so that the majority of people over the age of 70 need fewer than 7 hours of sleep each night. By this stage, the general quality of sleep may have be come lighter, with the proportion of deep sleep being reduced to approximately half an hour each night.

Chapter Two

The Nature of Sleep

In essence, sleep seems to involve nothing more than the act of closing our eyes and losing consciousness. This is because most of us regard the act of sleeping as a single, consistent experience, without realising that it involves, in fact, a complex series of contrasting phases of consciousness. Each phase has its order in the ideal sequence of a night's sleep, and its own purpose to perform.

Once we understand how these sequences of different quality sleep fit together, we are in a much better position to understand the mystery of sleep. As the saying goes, 'Knowledge is power' – this is especially true for any of us who feel at the mercy of unsatisfactory sleep patterns. Once we take the initial steps towards gaining a simple, working knowledge of what happens during those mysterious and elusive hours of slumber, we are in a stronger position to know how to take practical steps to rectify the situation.

Phases of Sleep

Rapid Eye Movement and Non-Rapid Eye Movement

A major watershed occurred in our understanding of sleep when the electro-encephalograph (EEG) was invented in the late 1920s. The invention of the EEG made it possible to pick up brain-wave activity and represent the findings in the form of lines that make decipherable patterns on a sheet of paper. With the study of EEGs, it became apparent that certain distinctive brain-wave patterns exist.

A further breakthrough came along in the mid-1950s, when it was discovered that something termed rapid eye movement sleep (REM sleep) occurs at regular intervals during sleep. Researchers observed that subjects' eyes started to move rapidly after roughly an hour's sleep although their eyes remained closed. They also noted that at this phase of rapid eye movement the subjects' EEG patterns were similar to those traced in conscious subjects. It became apparent that if subjects were woken during this phase of REM sleep, they would be able to recount especially vivid dreams.

As a consequence of these observations, the process of sleeping came to be divided into two forms: REM and non-REM sleep. From this point, a further division of quality of sleep became possible as it became clear that REM sleep itself could be separated into four distinct stages.

As a result of this work, we now know that in an average night's sleep an adult begins with Stage One: an initial phase of light sleep that is preceded by a sense of drowsiness and a drifting sensation. This is the phase of rest when some of us may find that we have what are called hypnogogic experiences such as a feeling of falling, glimpsing flashes of images, or the impression that someone is speaking to us.

This will predictably be followed by Stage Two: a deeper phase of sleep (traced by an EEG as wave sequences called 'sleep spindles'). By Stage Three, sleep has plunged into an even deeper phase, indicated by delta-wave activity, which is associated with especially relaxing properties. After we reach Stage Four (the most profoundly relaxing phase of sleep), we move back to Stage Three, followed by another phase of Stage Two.

This cycle is thought to last approximately 90 minutes or so, and after this comes the first short burst of REM activity. It may last anything between 5 and 15 minutes before the next four-stage cycle begins.

However, as our night's sleep progresses the phases of Stages Three and Four get progressively shorter, while the intermittent REM bursts get longer. It has been estimated that by the time we surface to consciousness in the morning, roughly a quarter of our time spent asleep will have been made up of REM sleep, while most of the rest will have been spent in Stage Two sleep.

Physical Changes that Occur in Sleep
When we are sinking into Stage One sleep, the process is associated with a drop in body temperature. As we descend into the deeper, progressively more relaxing stages of sleep, we experience a corresponding increase in physical indications of restfulness including slower patterns of breathing, lowered blood pressure and reduced heart rate.

However, physical responses in phases of REM sleep are quite a different story. As we enter a burst of REM sleep, brain-wave activity, heart rate, blood pressure and breathing rate begin to speed up, and may show signs of marked fluctuation. Blood flow to the brain is also noticeably increased during REM sleep. This escalating activity is accompanied by a paradoxical corresponding relaxation in muscle tension to a point that closely resembles a form of muscular paralysis. It has been suggested that this is the body's way of providing us with a clever 'restraining' mechanism that prevents us from acting out any destructive impulses that may be released during sleep.

The Importance of Balance

Because laboratory studies have shown that subjects deprived of REM sleep develop signs of obvious mental and emotional distress, it was initially thought that this was the most therapeutic phase of sleep. This conclusion was mistakenly reached when it was believed that the experience of dreaming was limited to time spent in REM sleep. Since dream-deprivation was thought to contribute to mental and emotional problems, the link between the importance of REM sleep and mental and emotional balance seemed clear.

However, it has since been established that we also spend some time dreaming in non-REM sleep. So, although it is accepted that time spent in REM sleep is essential for optimum mental and emotional health, it is now acknowledged that non-REM sleep also plays its own important part in keeping us emotionally and mentally healthy.

Particular benefits appear to be associated with Stage Four of non-REM sleep. It has been observed in people who require only a short sleep each night (five hours or less) that, although they may experience shorter phases of Stage One, Two and Three sleep, they need the average amount of Stage Four rest in order to stay well.

We have reached a point where we understand that the overall optimum balance of non-REM and REM sleep needs to be achieved if we are to gain maximum benefit from our hours of rest. Each of these two categories of sleep appears to bring special benefits, and neither appears to be able to make up for the loss of the other. So, as so in many other aspects of life, what we need essentially to be striving for in a healthy night's sleep is a state of overall balance and harmony.

Common Medical Conditions that Can Have a Negative Effect on Sleep

It is important to appreciate that the quality of sleep that we enjoy can be disturbed in the short or long term by suffering any of the conditions listed below. The situation may also be further complicated by the way in which some conventional drug treatments used to treat these conditions can have a significant impact on sleep duration, depth and pattern.

Anxiety

Anxiety and tension are two of the most powerful enemies of a sound, refreshing night's sleep. If we have been on mental and emotional 'red alert' most of the day, we are likely to find it extremely difficult to drift into a peaceful night's rest.

This is due to the body's in-built 'fight or flight' mechanism being triggered by stressful experiences during the day. If this reaction becomes a regular occurrence, our system will find it very difficult to relax mentally and physically, due to the raised levels of adrenalin circulating in our bodies.

Adrenalin is a powerful stress hormone that prepares our bodies to sprint away from or fight off any perceived threat or danger. As a result, heart rate speeds up, muscles receive extra blood supply, our senses function on a level of heightened sensitivity and alertness, while breathing naturally accelerates and becomes more shallow. Sadly, if these reactions become a frequent feature of daily life, we are likely to find that we experience escalating or persistent problems with high blood pressure, digestive disorders that fall under the general diagnostic term 'irritable bowel syndrome', physical, mental and emotional tension, and sleeplessness.

Unfortunately, anxiety symptoms of palpitations (consciousness of a rapid, fluttering heartbeat), mental and physical restlessness and panic can all have a tendency to be more severe at night. This may be partly due to the way that at night we do not have the benefit of the distractions of work or company that are available to us during the day.

If you suffer from anxiety, you may find that you either have immense difficulty drifting off to sleep, or that you fall asleep fairly quickly, only to find yourself waking with a jolt just an hour or two later. With this sort of frustrating pattern of sleeplessness you are likely to feel that you could sleep soundly for hours just before your alarm clock goes off.

However, it's not all bad news, since sleep problems of this kind are likely to respond very well to self-help measures that are known to benefit those of us who suffer from anxiety symptoms. These are discussed in Chapter Nine.

Depression

Poor or disturbed sleep patterns are one the major features of depression. There may not be so much of a tendency to find that it is difficult to get off to sleep (unless we experience a combination of anxiety that alternates with depression, which is quite common), but more that we wake in the early hours of the morning, usually feeling very mentally and emotionally low or jittery. When we are depressed, there can also be a tendency to want to 'nod off' at odd times during the day, partly as a result of the mental and emotional withdrawal that is so characteristic of depression, and sometimes as a consequence of the side-effects of conventional antidepressants which can sometimes lead to drowsiness.

It is not uncommon for anyone who suffers from depression to find that they develop a strong aversion to going to bed. This can be linked to a discernible pattern of mood, since depressive feelings are often most marked on first waking from sleep in the morning and tend to improve steadily as the day goes on. As a result, a dread of going to sleep can develop, since it is associated with waking up feeling very depressed.

At the other extreme, when clinical depression has reached a point where it is extremely distressing and severely disruptive to our quality of life, we may feel an instinctive desire to stay in bed for as long as possible. It's not uncommon when suffering from severe depression of this kind to want nothing more than to stay in bed all day with the duvet pulled over our heads. As you can imagine, if we get to this point and are sleeping fitfully during most of the day, we are likely to have even more difficulty achieving a sound night's rest.

Conventional antidepressant drugs may also have an impact on sleep quality, affecting the speed with which we enter the phases of sleep outlined above. We may also find that some antidepressants such as SSRIs may intensify episodes of particularly vivid dreaming or nightmares. In addition, it may take longer to pull ourselves around in the morning. This can be partly due to the condition itself, and partly due to taking antidepressant medication that has a sedative effect, such as one of the tricyclic drugs.

However, just as there are effective self-help measures that can be used to ease the troublesome symptoms of anxiety, we can also take effective, practical steps to break the pattern of mild to moderate depression-related sleep problems. These will be discussed in Chapter Nine.

Pre-Menstrual Syndrome (PMS)

Many women find that, apart from the notorious mood swings that are associated with PMS, one of the most irritating symptoms of this cyclical problem comes in the shape of wakefulness at night, which can be especially troublesome in the nights just preceding the onset of their period, or at mid-cycle when ovulation takes place.

This irritating tendency can be further aggravated by making unwise choices in what we eat and drink, since the cravings for sugar, chocolate, caffeine and alcohol that are a common feature of PMS bring their own problems in their wake. These can include jitteriness, severe changes of mood, fatigue and a lack of ability to drift off into a sound, relaxing sleep.

In addition, the hormonal fluctuations that are a natural part of a woman's menstrual cycle can also play their part in influencing the quality and pattern of sleep that we experience. It has been suggested that those of us who suffer regularly from noticeable symptoms of PMS may experience less REM and deep sleep than those of us who are fortunate enough to escape the problems of PMS.

If PMS is triggering problems with achieving a regular refreshing night's rest, it would be sensible to investigate stress-management techniques as an aid to effective relaxation. This has a particular relevance to easing problems related to hormone imbalance, since unmanaged stress appears to intensify problems of this kind.

This is partly due to the need for there to be an optimum balance in the body between stress hormones, such as adrenaline and cortisone, and the sex hormones oestrogen and progesterone if women are to experience optimum emotional, mental and physical health during their monthly cycles.

Poorly managed stress levels can also result in our taking refuge in negative coping strategies such as relying on cigarettes, alcohol and regular shots of caffeine in order to maintain the pace. As you will already have gathered, this is not good news for those who have problems switching off and dropping into a sound night's rest. Advice on the first steps towards learning to relax and unwind can be found in Chapter Nine.

The Menopause
As mentioned in the previous chapter, the transitional phase of the menopause can be a time when sleep disturbance comes sharply to the fore. Even women who escape problems with the common symptoms of hot flushes and/or night sweats may find that they flounder when it comes to having a refreshing, unbroken night's sleep.

This appears to be linked to fluctuations in the secretion of the sex hormones oestrogen and progesterone (as with similar problems in sleep disruption that occur at other major phases of hormonal fluctuation, such as PMS and during pregnancy).

This can be an especially frustrating situation, since it can have a marked effect in aggravating the diminished energy levels and mood swings that can also be associated with the menopause.

However dispiriting this may sound, it helps greatly to bear in mind that there are practical, proactive steps you can take to help cope with the situation. Perhaps the most important thing to bear in mind is that some menopausal symptoms such as disturbed sleep patterns, hot flushes and night sweats are characteristic of what is a transitory phase of development. In other words, once you have got through the menopause, you should find that you cease to experience these troublesome symptoms.

If sleeplessness is being aggravated by severe night sweats, you should seek professional medical help in order to deal with the problem. This can come from a conventional or alternative/complementary approach, depending on which feels appropriate. However, it may help at this point to mention that an alternative approach to treatment such as Western medical herbalism or homoeopathy will be aimed not merely at easing the night sweats, but also at re-establishing a healthy sleep pattern.

Overactive Thyroid Gland (Hyperthyroidism)
If you experience unexplained jitteriness, palpitations (conscious-

ness of a rapid or irregular heartbeat), weight loss, insomnia, rise in body temperature, an inability to switch off and physical restlessness, it's worth having a blood test done in order to check that you aren't suffering from an overactive thyroid. The result of a blood test is especially valuable in confirming or rejecting this diagnosis, since the symptoms of hyperthyroidism can sometimes be confused with a general anxiety state. As a result, an underlying, treatable condition may sometimes slip by undiagnosed.

Hyperthyroidism occurs when activity of the thyroid gland goes awry, resulting in too much of the hormonal secretion thyroxine being produced. Sometimes the whole thyroid gland may have gone into overdrive, or similar problems may be caused by the presence of a thyroid nodule.

It's helpful to know that this is a relatively rare disorder, and particularly rare in children. Those of us who are elderly and suffer from high blood pressure or hardening of the arteries may be more prone to hyperthyroidism. Once diagnosis is made, treatment may consist of any of the following options: taking anti-thyroid drugs, operating on the thyroid gland, or radioactive treatment targeted at the thyroid gland.

It has been suggested that more Stage Three and Stage Four deep sleep is needed if we suffer from hyperthyroidism in order to benefit fully from a night's rest.

ME (Myalgic Encephalomyelitis)

It is only comparatively recently that ME has been recognised as a serious illness, as a result of the findings of a recent British Government report. Previously, this condition was frequently dismissed as a psychosomatic problem (in other words, 'all in the mind'), and there are still some reservations on the part of some conventional doctors about the nature of this illness. This slightly confusing situation is further compounded by the absence of any definitive test that can confirm a diagnosis of ME.

As a result, the conclusion is often reached that ME is likely to be the problem when other medical conditions with similar symptoms have been ruled out (such as an underactive thyroid gland). This tendency to reach a negative diagnosis is not unique to ME, since other chronic conditions such as irritable bowel syndrome are often diagnosed when tests have ruled out the possibility of other medical conditions that are known to affect the digestive tract, such as a stomach ulcer or the presence of parasites or thread worms.

Common symptoms of ME are wide-ranging, and may include any of the following: overwhelming exhaustion, difficulty concentrating, bouts of perspiration, palpitations, recurrent headaches, depression, anxiety, poor co-ordination, muscle aches and sleep disturbance. The general sleep quality of ME patients appears to be adversely affected by their tendency to produce alpha-type waves that are associated with relaxed wakefulness, rather than the theta waves that should be present in Stage One sleep or the delta waves that are indicative of deep sleep.

No one knows for a fact what triggers this perplexing illness, but certain common factors appear to be shared by those patients who suffer from the problem. Damaged immune system performance, severe viral illness at a time of marked stress and an adverse reaction to vaccinations may all be predisposing factors to developing ME.

Sleep problems are a particularly upsetting aspect of ME, since the profound mental, emotional and physical exhaustion that are the hallmarks of this condition are made even more overwhelming if good-quality, refreshing sleep proves to be elusive on a regular basis.

From a conventional medical standpoint, this problem can be eased by prescribing a small dose of the antidepressant amitriptyline, which has sedative-like properties. This can break the negative cycle of restlessness and wakefulness at night, and should not lead to drowsiness on first waking, as can be caused by higher doses of this medication.

However, it is important to bear in mind that alternative and complementary medicines have a particularly positive and practical role to play in supporting those who suffer from ME. A gentle, graded exercise regime that incorporates yoga, aromatherapy massage, nutritional guidance, homoeopathy, osteopathy, cranial osteopathy and manual lymphatic drainage can all play a part in gently relieving the broad spectrum of ME symptoms, including poor-quality sleep.

Since ME is a chronic condition (well established and likely to involve repeated, acute flare-ups of symptoms), the most effective alternative and complementary treatment is likely to be obtained from a trained practitioner in any of the therapies mentioned above.

Snoring
This is often not so much a problem for the sufferer, but for the part-

ner who sleeps with them! There's nothing quite so disruptive of a heavenly deep sleep than extended loud bursts of snoring coming from the other side of the bed. If the problem is very severe, it can be so bad that the snorer actually wakes him- or herself up as well.

Simple measures that may improve the situation can include any of the following:

- Weight loss: since being significantly overweight can exaggerate the problem (as well as bringing a potential host of additional health problems in its wake), heavy snorers should consider taking up a healthy, sensible weight-loss plan.
- If catarrhal congestion or allergies are contributing to the problem, consider consulting an alternative or complementary therapist. Good therapies to consider would include Western medical herbalism, homoeopathy, naturopathy, nutritional medicine or traditional Chinese medicine.
- Nasal strips, which gently hold the nostrils open, can be expensive as a long-term strategy, but they do seem to help some sufferers. They can be especially worth while if snoring is only a major problem when associated with cold symptoms.
- Getting into the habit of sleeping on your side rather than your back also appears to be a simple way of reducing a tendency to snore. The occasional kick from an irate partner can often give the necessary impetus to move into the correct position!

Sleep Apnoea

This is a distressing condition that is becoming more widely publicised. Associated with loud snoring, breath-holding and choking spasms through the night, it has been identified as a condition that can be associated with a number of significant health risks. These include an increased risk of sleepiness during the day, strokes, heart disease and high blood pressure. Sufferers of sleep apnoea are also likely to experience mood swings, persistent fatigue and a diminished interest in sex.

If you suspect you may have a problem with this condition, it's worth seeking the advice of your GP, who may suggest you use a nasal mask at night. Called a continuous positive airway pressure device (CPAP), it is strapped to the face during sleep and acts by ensuring that the air passages are kept open. In addition, it's also worth employing some of the self-help measures listed above for snoring problems.

Restless Leg Syndrome

This is a term used to describe a maddening sensation that usually sets in at night and which leads to a compulsion to keep changing the position of your legs. Possible sensations include a persistent crawling or tingling feeling in the legs, or simply a feeling that it's impossible to keep the lower limbs still. Those who tend towards disturbed sleep, who are easily woken, or who find it very difficult to get to sleep will find restless leg syndrome an almost impossible problem to deal with.

There is no definitive treatment on offer, but any of the following measures may be of help:
- Taking gentle, regular exercise such as walking can do a great deal to support efficient circulation in the legs. Although restless leg syndrome is not thought to be related specifically to circulation problems, the legs are generally going to feel in better condition when regular exercise is taken. Walking is even more beneficial if varicose veins are an additional complication.
- If symptoms are aggravated during or just after phases of high stress levels, it's worth employing some basic relaxation strategies. These may include soaking in a warm bath scented with soothing essential oils before retiring, or using a relaxation technique that focuses on letting go of tension in specific muscle groups.
- If problems with restless leg syndrome are established and severe, it's definitely worth consulting an alternative or complementary health practitioner from any of the disciplines mentioned above.
- Check how much caffeine you take in an average day. (If you're not sure about the relative caffeine content in various drinks, see the caffeine content table in Chapter Five.) Anyone who drinks more than two cups of coffee a day should consider cutting down, since caffeine appears to contribute to an aggravation of generalised symptoms of stress, in addition to making it harder for us to switch off at night. As we can see, a high caffeine intake wouldn't be doing anyone who suffers from restless leg syndrome any favours.
- If problems with restless legs have become severe or well estab-

lished and you haven't had a blood test for a while to check iron levels, it's worth doing so. This is because iron deficiency may contribute to this irritating problem.

- Consider taking a good-quality multimineral supplement, since low calcium or magnesium levels may aggravate restless leg syndrome.

Chapter Three

Sleep and the Mind

Sleep deprivation that goes on for an extended period of time can have a severe negative impact on your state of mental and emotional equilibrium. It's not uncommon to find that severe problems with sleeplessness can leave you feeling indecisive, moody, irritable and generally jittery and anxious.

This is thought to be partly due to the way in which the process of dreaming allows us to release material from the subconscious that we can explore safely through our dreams. Although many of us won't remember the details of our dreams on waking (some of us may just be aware of their general mood, unless our memories are jogged by something that happens the following day), they do appear to play a significant role in helping us maintain psychological balance.

The Royal Road to the Unconscious: The Importance of Dreams

Dreams have mysterious and fascinating qualities that have preoccupied human beings for centuries. In the ancient world, dreams were used to predict the future, and the Greeks used them as an instrument to heal the sick.

Things became even more interesting with regard to the interpretation of dreams at the beginning of the 20th century. This was the period when the burgeoning field of psychoanalysis was initiated by Sigmund Freud and dreams took on a new significance. It was Freud who referred to dreaming as 'the royal road to the unconscious'.

He regarded the seemingly random events that occur in our dreams as the coded or disguised expression of our unconscious desires. Freud asserted that these drives would be kept out of contact with our conscious minds due to their 'unacceptable' nature. 'Unacceptable' can be regarded from Freud's perspective as usually being connected to either unbridled aggression or sexual desire.

Our dreams allow us to acknowledge and work through our preoccupations and desires. And although the symbolism of dreams generally eludes the dreamer, Freud believed that with the help of a psychoanalyst the symbolism of a dream could be interpreted or 'translated' into its original meaning. As a result, it would be possible through psychoanalysis to gain a greater understanding of what might be going on in the subconscious mind.

A contrasting spin on this psychoanalytical perspective was provided by Carl Jung, who disagreed strongly with Freud over the significance and value of our dreams. Jung argued that the activity of dreaming is a way of balancing out whatever aspects of our lives are being neglected in the way we consciously live our lives. Or, looked at from another angle, he believed that our dreams form part of the spectrum of continuous 24-hour mental activity that takes place each day.

So, from Jung's perspective, rather than being an escape route for subversive desires, dreams play a positive role in bringing overlooked aspects of our personalities and characters to our attention. Unlike Freud, Jung argued that this process is an end in itself, and only requires exploration through analysis if we begin to show signs of becoming mentally or emotionally imbalanced.

As suggested in the previous chapter, it was originally thought that dreaming was limited to bursts of REM activity. However, we now know that while REM dreams have a characteristically vivid form and nature, we also dream during other phases of sleep.

We appear most of the time to dream in colour, and most experiences are visual in nature rather than auditory. During the light phases of sleep as we are drifting off, we are likely to experience hypnagogic states that are not quite fully fledged dreams. These are common to the experience of dozing and are short lived and more subject to our conscious control. In this state we may also think we can hear voices.

Nightmares can occur in a phase of sleep that is distinct from REM activity. Night terrors in children seem most likely to happen in Stage Four deep sleep, while anxiety dreams in adults are more likely to be reported as the sleeper wakes from REM sleep. Talking in sleep is most likely to happen in Stage Two non-REM sleep, while those of us who sleepwalk will do so in Stage Four of deep sleep.

However complex all of this appears to be, one point comes through loud and clear: we need to sleep refreshingly and dream each night if we are to have the best chance of attaining mental clarity and emotional balance.

Apart from the emotional benefits of dreaming each night, there is also a strikingly practical role to be played by a healthy sleep and dreaming pattern. This is linked to the problem-solving potential of sleeping and dreaming, which can be quite mind-boggling at times. Many of us have had the experience of grappling unsuccessfully with a problem with our conscious minds in our waking hours, only to discover that the solution is presented to us in our dreams, or springs into our minds as we wake.

Capturing the Ephemeral: Recording Dreams

We all appear to dream when we are asleep, but memories of our dreams are very fleeting. As a result, unless we make a note of the subject matter of our dreams as we wake, we are likely to find it extremely difficult to recall them.

It has been suggested that we may begin to understand a little more about what makes us tick mentally and emotionally if we pay attention to and explore any recurring or persistent themes that appear in our dreams. If we do this, we are likely to discover that, while many of our dreams are made up of nothing more than seemingly random images that may have been sparked off by the events of an average day, there are other, strikingly persistent themes that surface when we are feeling short-term anxiety, depression or insecurity.

If we establish that this is the case, we may begin to pay more attention to ourselves at times like these, cutting ourselves more mental and emotional slack if we need it, and finding positive ways of self-help in order to support ourselves through demanding or difficult times.

If the idea of exploring your dream-life is appealing, the following will help you recall regular themes that appear each night:

- Keep a note pad and pen near your bedside so you can jot down a few notes as you wake.
- If it's difficult to capture the mood of a dream or series of dreams in words, sketch a few key images instead. They will still serve as a

reminder and this is true even if your artistic skills leave a lot to be desired!

- Make a note of the main mood of your dream and your emotional response to it.
- It may help to date each night's jottings, so that the order and frequency with which certain themes appear can be distinguished. For this to be most illuminating, it will also help to make a note of how you were feeling in general during your waking hours (for example, stressed, relaxed, upset or excited).

Don't be discouraged if at first there seems to be no rhyme or reason to the substance of your dreams. It may take a very long time of recording them before you begin to observe anything that seems meaningful.

Practical Measures to Help You Prepare for Sleep

Although some of the following will appear to be simple common sense, these measures can be immensely helpful in preparing you for a refreshing night's sleep and preventing you from falling into some common counter-productive habits. Try to incorporate these positive strategies at times of tension as basic stress-busting measures. You are likely to find it's well worth the effort!

- Always refrain from doing any stimulating mental work for at least a couple of hours before retiring, otherwise you are likely to find switching off an extremely frustrating and elusive experience.
- If a guided relaxation technique or a specific meditation exercise doesn't appeal, make a point of doing something that feels conducive to unwinding instead. This could involve, for example, listening to favourite pieces of music or reading a novel.
- Make a point of having a night-time ritual that your mind and body can recognise as a preparation for sleep. This shouldn't be so rigid that it becomes part of an inflexible routine, but should have recognisable boundaries so that mind and body can be alerted to the fact that it's time to start winding down. Simple examples of this sort of activity include having a warm bath, doing a facial massage routine, cleaning your teeth or doing a breathing exercise. Once they become familiar, these will serve

as signals that it's time for your mind and body to relax and let go.

- Avoid watching television in bed, however seductive it might seem. WatchingTV has a dual drawback since it tends to stimulate the mind rather than encouraging it to move into restful mode, and the associated postural problems can contribute to stress-related symptoms such as tension headaches.

In his self-help sleep guide entitled *Restful Sleep*, Deepak Chopra suggests that we should rethink our response to lying awake and not being able to drift off peacefully to sleep. It's certainly true that many of us may instinctively find ourselves becoming progressively tense, anxious and despairing as we lie in bed wide awake. What Deepak Chopra suggests is adopting a perspective of 'not minding'. In other words, instead of lying there fretting about not yet having drifted off to sleep, you should try to accept that you are awake at that point and consciously relax your body as much as possible. It has certainly been my own experience that once this state of gentle acceptance is reached, and you begin to appreciate that you are still enjoying the positive benefits of rest as you lie in bed, you are likely to find when you wake up several hours' later that you have unexpectedly and peacefully drifted off to sleep.

The Importance of Guided Relaxation

Becoming familiar with practising a step-by-step relaxation exercise has particular benefits in the sleep department which go beyond its general stress-reducing effect on mind, emotions and body.

This is due to the way that regular practice of a guided relaxation technique switches on a state of mind and body that has been called 'the relaxation response'. Regular, conscious induction of this 'chilled-out' state encourages the parasympathetic nervous system to come into play. This mode of response is characterised by reduced oxygen consumption, decreased heart rate, slower respiration and a measurable lowering of blood lactate levels. If we consider that respiration and heart rate are slowed down in the profoundly restful stage of deep sleep, we can see that there are obvious similarities between the results of the relaxation response and the physiological effects of restful sleep.

As a result, regular practice of a relaxation technique (such as those described in Chapter Nine) can go a long way towards effectively preparing us for a restful night's sleep. Granted, there are also significant differences between a state of profound relaxation and deep sleep (for instance, the presence of alpha waves is a common indication of a relaxed state of mind and body, while alpha waves are not, as a rule, present in sleep). Nevertheless, learning an effective, guided relaxation technique and taking time out to practise it each day will give us a better chance of switching off at night.

Effective relaxation is just one of the foundation stones of a good night's sleep, as you will discover in the next chapter, which explores additional practical steps you can take to make your bedroom a sleep-inducing sanctuary.

Chapter Four

Preparing the Body for Sleep

There are many practical steps you can take in order to ensure that you are as physically relaxed as possible in preparation for a refreshing night's sleep. The scope of the information that follows is deliberately broad, and attempts to be genuinely holistic in its approach. By becoming as imaginative along these lines as possible, you are likely to find that there are surprising allies at your disposal that you may never have considered before. Be prepared the strategies explored below are a far cry from being limited to finding alternatives to conventional sleeping tablets (though these aren't neglected, either, and are discussed in Chapter Eight).

Evaluating the Context

It's sometimes so easy to neglect the obvious, and overlooking the nature of the surroundings in which you attempt to enjoy a good night's rest is no exception. You may be enthusiastically paying attention to the way you eat and drink and how much exercise you take, making sure you meditate each day and trying alternative medical self-help, only to find that sleep is proving frustratingly elusive.

If this is the case, it's definitely worth taking a moment to evaluate objectively the sleep-inducing or sleep-disturbing qualities of your bedroom. Always remember that surroundings can often unwittingly reflect our state of mind. If you consider that the state your bedroom is in will be the last image you see before you close your eyes, and the first you see on waking, it's not really too fanciful to suggest that your surroundings can play a significant role in the quality of sleep you enjoy.

The following advice has been designed to provide a realistic over view of the basic requirements of a restful, healthy sleeping environment. Always remember these are general practical hints to be applied in ways that appeal to your individual tastes. After all, it's your bedroom and, above all else, you need to feel relaxed and happy with the results!

Transforming Your Bedroom into a Sleep-inducing Sanctuary

- Reduce the clutter!

A bedroom filled with objects, papers, clothes and other items that haven't been put away can, without your realising it, reinforce any feelings of anxiety, powerlessness or dissatisfaction that may be pre-occupying you. Clutter-clearing is one of the basic principles of Feng Shui, since it is thought that heaps of unnecessary objects on the floor will block the flow of vital energy around us. Even if the idea of balancing the flow of vital energy is a bit too esoteric for you, on a purely practical level, removing clutter by putting items away into cupboards or wardrobes can feel enormously therapeutic. It can feel even more exhilarating and liberating to throw away any items that you aren't sentimentally attached to, or that have outstayed their welcome.

- Pay attention to the amount of tranquillity you enjoy each night.

If your bedroom overlooks or is near a busy street, the noise level that continues late into the night and begins early each morning is unlikely to make for a refreshing night's rest. Consider moving the position of your bedroom (for instance to the back of the house or flat, which might be more peaceful) or, if this isn't practical, consider investing in some effective double-glazing in order to provide a buffer against any unwelcome disturbance overnight.

- Keep it dark.

Much as we are likely to appreciate and benefit from well-lit surroundings during the day, our requirements during the hours of sleep are quite another matter. Ideally you need curtains or blinds that are dark enough to filter out any light that will prevent you from drifting off into a sound sleep at night, and that allow you to continue sleeping after dawn. On the other hand, always avoid the mistake of going for extra-thick 'black-out' curtains, which have the disadvantage of making it very difficult to wake easily in the morning.

- Colour me sleepy.

When choosing a colour scheme for a bedroom, obviously the most important thing is the element of personal taste. Having said this, it can be helpful to know that certain colours have a reputation for enhancing certain moods and atmospheres. A lot of the discussion around the therapeutic effect of specific colour tones can appear to come down to little more than common sense (for instance, bright red is stimulating and energy-enhancing), but it can be interesting to consider this perspective when you are considering the merits of certain shades over others. Blue is regarded as soothing and calming, green shades are said to be mood-balancing, while yellow is uplifting and crimson colours are thought to be best reserved for rooms where we may feel we need an energy boost. While indigo is unlikely to be used in large quantities because it's such a strong shade, the presence of small amounts in a softer version (for instance in the form of cushions or a throw) is considered to be conducive to meditation and contemplation.

- Fresh air

Ventilation also plays its part in contributing to or interfering with a sound night's sleep. Try to make sure that the bedroom is neither too hot and stuffy, nor so chilly that it feels uncomfortable. In spring and summer, fresh air from an open window can feel very welcome overnight in order to prevent the bedroom feeling muggy, but those who suffer from hay fever may do better with an electric fan. This should be placed at a strategic place, not too near the bed, otherwise that you may feel uncomfortably chilled in the middle of the night.

- Allergic reactions

If allergies, rhinitis, eczema or asthma are an established problem, going to bed can become a less than attractive protect if you know you are going to sneeze, itch or wheeze as soon as your head hits the pillow. Practical measures should include avoiding pillows and duvets made from feathers, opting instead for fibre-filled versions. When buying these, it's always worth asking the shop assistant if the product you are buying is suitable for anyone who suffers from any of the problems mentioned above. In addition, use mattress and pillow covers that can be easily slipped off and laundered frequently. Those who are allergic to house dust mites also need to hoover and dust frequently and diligently, in order to minimise contact with the droppings of these ubiquitous mites. If contact with detergent residue tends to spark off problems with allergic reactions, always make a point of rinsing bed linen twice over in order to ensure that any traces of soap powder are removed.

- Bedclothes

Choosing whether to opt for a duvet or blankets and sheets is really down to individual taste. Those who strongly dislike being hemmed in at night are likely to react negatively to the sheet-and-blanket approach and those who prefer a light but cosy bed environment are most likely going to choose to sleep under a duvet. Some of us may like to ring the changes according to the season, opting for the warmth of blankets during the winter, and changing to a feather-light duvet with the warmth of late spring and summer.

- Your mattress

If you seem to be tossing and turning endlessly in search of a comfortable position in bed, ask yourself how old your mattress is. Without realising it, we can sometimes end up sleeping on a mattress that has long ago passed its sell-by date. The average life-span of a mattress should be no more than eight to ten years maximum: tell-tale signs include lumps, bumps and any signs of sagging in other words, the general signs of ageing! When investing in a new bed or replacement mattress, mention any special needs (such as back pain or allergies) you may have to the salesperson, since he or she should be trained to advise you on the best purchase to suit your health profile and your budget.

- Pillow talk

Be imaginative when it comes to buying pillows, especially if tension headaches or neck and back pain are a problem. Possibilities to choose from include custom-made pillows that are designed to keep the neck in optimum alignment, to large, square continental pillows that provide excellent support when sitting up in bed. Ideally the support given from pillows and mattresses should be firm but not so hard that they feel uncomfortable. Although sinking into a soft pillow and mattress may initially feel blissful, in time this may be counter-productive, since they don't provide you with the necessary support for your neck and spine.

- Nightwear

Again, this is very much down to individual taste, lifestyle and the season. For those who favour the Marilyn Monroe approach of wearing nothing but a favourite perfume (or aftershave for men) all year round, there really isn't an issue here! Others may love to wear sexy nightwear, while the bedsock and nightshirt may be more at a premium for anyone who hates being cold in bed. As a general rule, whatever nightwear is chosen needs to feel comfortable and to be as unrestrictive as possible, so it's good to avoid anything too tight around the neck or waist, or anything that has a tendency to bunch up during a restless night. The best fabrics for inducing a good night's rest are those that naturally allow the skin to breathe (silk for the sensually inclined, cotton for the more Spartan). Because artificial fibres tend to hold heat in and create a significant amount of static electricity, nightwear made from these is often not the best choice for contributing to a sound night's rest, especially on a muggy summer's night.

- Using an ioniser

If waking sometimes feels traumatic, leaving you feeling grouchy, muzzy-headed and groggy, it's worth considering investing in an ioniser that can sit on a bedside table. The benefits of using an ioniser are thought to come about as a result of balancing the negative and positive ions in the atmosphere. When the balance tips in favour of positive ions we may feel headachy and fatigued, while increasing the negative ions appears to make us feel generally clear-headed and relaxed.

- Wake-up call

If you find waking to the shrill ringing or buzzing of an alarm clock a strain each morning, consider a gentler incentive to waking. There are a number of different designs of alarm clock on the market, including ones that use a slowly increasing light to mimic the effect of dawn. Some versions come complete with recordings of birdsong if you want the full effect.

Simple Advice for Shift-workers

Those in jobs that require working antisocial hours are especially at risk of poor, unrefreshing sleep patterns. The problem can be made more intense if the shifts change on a regular basis, so that you don't even get the chance of getting into the habit of a regular, if unconventional, daytime-to-nighttime rhythm.

Problems that can occur as a result of working shifts include recurrent fatigue, emotional strain with a tendency to snap easily, diminished co-ordination and reduced levels of concentration. This may be partly connected to the way in which sleep patterns alter as result of shift-work. Although those who are used to shift-work sleep for proportionally longer periods of time, the balance of phases of sleep will be different to those experienced by those of us who sleep regularly at night. Shift-workers have been shown to enjoy less REM sleep and linger longer in light sleep, and they tend to experience a lighter, more fitful quality of rest. The cumulative result of these changes in sleep pattern and sleep quality is that you are likely to feel less refreshed on waking.

Some people may have constitutions that cope more easily with the pressures involved in shift-work than others, but the following advice will be helpful to anyone who faces this particular challenge:

- Incorporate regular exercise into your lifestyle in order to help diminish stress levels and improve all-round fitness. For a quick run-down of appropriate options, see pages 56-61 later in this chapter.
- If your sleep pattern has gone through a difficult phase, make a point of reducing or cutting out alcohol intake. This really does have a beneficial effect on sleep quality as a whole. On no account take a drink before going to work, since it's likely to exaggerate all of the problems associated with shift-work listed above.
- If you benefit from a quick snooze and find it refreshing, take a 'power' nap before beginning your shift. This should obviously be avoided by anyone who finds napping a counter-productive, drowsiness-inducing experience.
- Some people may be able to have a full-spectrum light box installed at work; this may help to stimulate a balanced mood and general sense of increased energy and alertness.
- Follow the advice given earlier in this chapter to establish the most harmonious, relaxing sleeping environment.
- Anyone who needs to take conventional medication on a regular basis should consult his or her GP about the optimum time to take this medication. This is especially important where sedative medication is involved.

Breathing Techniques to Relax Body and Mind

We all tend to take breathing for granted unless we encounter problems such as a bout of wheezing or a panic attack. It's only at times like these, when our breathing becomes laboured or anxious, that we realise how essential effortless respiration is to our sense of well-being.

The reason we tend to be unaware of our breathing patterns is that the activity of inhaling oxygen and exhaling carbon dioxide is classed as an involuntary activity. In other words, however essential it might be to staying alive, we don't have to concentrate on the process of respiration in order for it to continue fairly smoothly.

The problem is that, without our realising it, our breathing patterns generally reflect how stressed or relaxed we feel, since we tend to adopt a particular pattern of breathing when we are under pressure. The common reaction to feeling tense involves a tendency to breathe rapidly and in a shallow way, using only a small proportion of our lung capacity. If this goes on for long enough, it leads to the unpleasant sensations of hyperventilation associated with severe anxiety states.

Unfortunately, if you are unaware of the breathing patterns we adopt in response to phases of strain and tension, you can unwittingly make the situation worse. If you get caught in this vicious circle you are likely to find that relaxing and unwinding moves progressively further and further beyond your reach. This is because taking quick, short breaths from your upper chest has an adverse effect on the balance between the blood gases oxygen and carbon dioxide in your bloodstream.

An unfortunate side-effect of this imbalance is an increase in feelings of anxiety, palpitations and light-headedness. You may also begin to feel a tingling sensation in your arms and hands, which is likely to increase your sense of panic. As a result you are likely to breathe even more quickly and unevenly, and so the unfortunate loop of anxious breathing goes on.

The solution to this distressing cycle lies within your grasp, and is simplicity itself. It involves using controlled, relaxing breathing techniques that have the positive effect of clearing your mind while having a rapid, profoundly calming effect on your mind and body. Since these techniques have include such a tranquillity-inducing and mood-balancing effect, they can be of particular benefit when used as an effective preparation for a sound night's sleep.

Not only does regular practice of the relaxing breathing technique outlined below encourage your mind to switch off, but it can also help induce a powerful sensation of physical relaxation. As a result, you are less likely to suffer from muscle tension, cramps or twitchy legs as you are ready to fall asleep.

Basic Steps

This is a technique often used as part of the practice of yoga called diaphragmatic breathing. It involves learning to take gentle, conscious breaths that bring the diaphragm (the large sheet of flexible muscle that lies at the bottom of the chest cavity) into our conscious control.

It's easier to establish that the diaphragm is being called into play if you gently rest one hand on your abdomen, just above your navel. When you have mastered this effective, tension-busting breathing technique, you will have an effective tool at your disposal that you can use any time you feel stressed or anxious.

It's worth taking a moment to learn how different this form of breathing feels in contrast to the shallow, fast breaths you may be used to taking.

1. Sit in a high-backed chair that gives adequate support to your spine and discourages slouching or hunching over. Poor postural habits of this kind have a negative effect on breathing by restricting the amount of air you can take in. If lying down feels more appealing (and especially if using this technique as part of your preparations for sleep), lie down on a firm surface making sure that the surrounding temperature is warm enough. Always bear in mind that the act of relaxation tends to involve a drop in body temperature; as a result, always prepare for effective relaxation by being warmly and comfortably dressed.
2. Take a moment to focus your attention on your breathing before slowly filling your lungs with air as you breathe gently and steadily in. As your lungs fully inflate from the top to the base, the hand you have on your abdomen should slowly rise a little upwards and outwards.
3. Pause for a second before slowly emptying your lungs from the base to the top as you fully and steadily exhale. You will know this is happening as you notice the hand resting on your abdomen move back to its starting position.

4. If you feel comfortable with how this feels, take another five breaths in this way before pausing and resuming your normal breathing pattern. If you experience any uneasiness, light-headedness or dizziness, stop, resuming only when you feel ready to do so.

Once you feel familiar with this relaxing breathing technique, you can use it whenever you feel tense, stressed, anxious or under pressure. The very act of focusing on the way in which you are breathing can be enough to break a negative cycle of anxiety, since you will feel you can take some positive action to change how you are feeling. The very feeling of helplessness that accompanies an episode of anxiety can make the anxious feelings worse. The knowledge that you have an effective tool at your disposal that instantly helps you feel less tense can do a great deal to liberate you from feelings of apprehension that can have the undesirable knock-on effect of making a poor-quality sleep pattern worse.

As you become more familiar with breathing in this controlled, relaxed way, you can dispense with the additional help of lying down or putting your hand on your abdomen: these are just props to help the beginner establish that he or she is doing this calming breathing technique correctly. As a result, you can use this form of breathing in any situation where you feel you need it, without there being any visual clues to what you are doing. This could apply to any pressurised situation, from a fraught boardroom confrontation to receiving a difficult phone call or lying awake in the early hours of the morning.

There are important additional benefits that spring from this calming method of breathing. They include increased clarity of mind, enhanced capacity to focus, greater decisiveness and improved mental and physical energy levels.

Bathing and Hydrotherapy Techniques to Enhance Good-quality Sleep

Many of us may feel that we would love to spend some time at a health spa luxuriating in treatments that are reputed to make us feel relaxed, rejuvenated or energised, depending on our individual needs and requirements. Unfortunately, escaping to a blissful spa resort is expensive and time-consuming, and as a result may seem out of our reach.

However, taking time to pamper yourself is neither indulgent nor unreasonable. By looking after yourself you can make a significant impact on whether you enjoy high-quality health that allows you to roll with whatever punches life may throw at you or tend to fall at the first hurdle due to lack of emotional, mental and physical resilience.

The good news is that pampering yourself needn't be expensive or involve days away from home. Basic hydrotherapy and massage techniques can be incorporated into your regular routine not slavishly, but as something to look forward to as a valuable opportunity to rest and recharge your mind and body. Most of the simple steps below can also be used as excellent groundwork for a refreshing night's sleep.

Water has incredible therapeutic powers that can be used to energise or relax us. Many people instinctively feel that water can have a profound effect on how they feel (for instance, soaking in a warm bath at the end of a taxing day, or getting into a brisk shower to kick-start the day when we need to be bright-eyed and bushy-tailed).

Apart from these very basic applications of hydrotherapy, you can enjoy further benefits once you are aware of the techniques you can employ to enhance a state of mental and physical relaxation, or to give yourself a much-needed energy boost. The measures outlined below are included with a view to being practical, accessible and, above all, pleasurable. The importance of the latter should never be lost sight of in any programme that seeks to boost your basic levels of health and vitality. Making some of these simple hydrotherapy techniques part of your life is going to become something you look forward to, rather than a chore that you will want to put off.

Bathing for Relaxation

Although bathing is hardly going to be an unusual experience for you, conditions are not often conducive to making the sensation the totally unwinding pleasure it can be. Pressures of time, demands of young children putting a bath off until last thing at night when all you want to do is roll into bed can all contribute to making bath time a rushed pursuit. As a result, you are likely to emerge from the bath hot, bothered and flustered rather than renewed and relaxed. The following hints may help in changing this.

- Temperature control

Avoid taking baths that are extremely hot, since these can make you feel enervated and exhausted rather than pleasantly relaxed. This is partly due to the way in which very hot baths put extra strain on the heart and circulatory system. From a purely cosmetic point of view, they also have a disastrous effect on skin tone, exaggerating sagging skin, broken veins, cellulite and blotchiness. Make a point of having a leisurely soak in water that is pleasantly warm instead.

- Make your bathroom a place that is conducive to relaxation.

Choose colours for the walls that are soothing and calming, and opt for complementary colours when choosing towels and bath accessories. In this way you will be able to carry the tranquil mood through and create a total effect.

- Use scented candles.

These can play a large effect in establishing the atmosphere you are after. Flickering candlelight in the bathroom can encourage relaxation by its very soft and gentle nature, while the addition of essential oils can further enhance the soothing and sensual experience. Always follow simple, precautionary safety measures when using candles: burn them in a suitable, heat-resistant holder (this is of particular importance if your bath is made of acrylic, since this can be damaged by contact with heat); never leave lit candles to burn unattended; avoid moving or carrying a candle once it has been lit; take care to trim candle wicks regularly in order to ensure that the flame burns steadily at a safe height.

- Avoid jumping into a hot bath after eating a heavy meal.

This can lead to indigestion and insomnia. Always make a point of leaving an interval of at least two to three hours after eating a large meal before bathing. For foods and drinks that help induce sound sleep (and those that have the opposite, adverse effect), see Chapter Five. Vigorous exercise should also be avoided just prior to taking a hot bath, for similar reasons.

Relaxing Bath Suggestions

The practical use of aromatherapy essential oils to help you unwind (this will include suggestions for preparing a soothing aromatherapy soak) will be discussed in Chapter Eight. Meanwhile, the following alternatives can help you with ideas for some basic de-stressing bath options.

Epsom Salt Soak
This is an excellent strategy to try if you've been living in the fast lane for a while and are painfully aware that, as a consequence, you've been eating and drinking unwisely and generally pushing yourself too hard. Indulging in the occasional Epsom salt bath, followed by an early night, is an excellent first step to detoxing and getting yourself back on track.

- Dissolve 2 cups of Epsom salts in a comfortably warm bath and immerse yourself for up to 20 minutes, or a shorter period if you begin to feel too hot. The bath water can be topped up in order to maintain a steady level of heat.

This form of bathing will induce a marked sweat, as toxins are eliminated through the pores of the skin. Once you are out, wrap up snugly and get into a comfortably warm bed.

You may find that your skin is drier than usual the next day, so do make a point of applying a good-quality body lotion to moisturise thoroughly any areas that are showing signs of dryness.

Caution
Anyone who suffers from high blood pressure or skin conditions such as eczema should give Epsom salt bathing a miss. If in doubt consult your doctor or pharmacist.

Dead Sea Salt Treatment
Dead Sea salts can also provide a relaxing, detoxifying experience at the end of a stressful day. As a treatment, the minerals to be found in Dead Sea salts appear to speed up the body's capacity for excreting toxins and encouraging the efficient turnover of surface skin cells which may be contributing to a dull or uneven skin tone. This process can be further encouraged by skin brushing or exfoliating with a commercially prepared cream or gel skin scrub before bathing. (If you are new to the idea of dry skin brushing, details of this naturopathic technique can be found on page 51.)

- Add 3 or 4 handfuls of Dead Sea salts to a comfortably warm bath, swirling the water around until they are dissolved. Soak for approximately 10 minutes, or as long as feels comfortable.

Once out of the bath, shower off the salts and apply lashings of body lotion before relaxing in a warm bed.

Caution
As with Epsom salts, Dead Sea salt bathing should not be undertaken by anyone with high blood pressure or skin conditions such as eczema. If in doubt about its advisability, seek medical advice.

Seaweed Baths
Seaweed and seawater are thought to have powerful therapeutic properties, supporting and encouraging the body's in-built capacity for cleansing and excreting toxic waste.
- Add the recommended amount of powdered seaweed to a warm bath, making sure that the water isn't too hot. It's especially important to check this, since bathing in too hot a seaweed bath can trigger unpleasant sensations of palpitations and agitation. Soak for a minimum of 10 minutes and a maximum of 20, making sure to step into a warm shower afterwards in order to wash off any residue of seaweed. Wrap up in warm dressing gown before retiring.

Dry Skin Brushing
- Use a long-handled, natural firm-bristle brush that allows you to make long, sweeping strokes. Brush in smooth, rhythmical movements, starting from the feet and moving progressively upwards from the lower legs to the thighs and hips. Once the lower body has been covered in sweeping brush strokes, move your attention to the upper half, moving in a downwards direction this time towards your heart. The pressure used should be firm enough to give the skin a glowing, pinkish appearance, but not so hard that it feels sore or uncomfortable. Never dry skin brush any patches of broken skin, eczema, psoriasis, or broken or varicose veins.

Hydrotherapy Wraps
The following techniques may be used occasionally to relax the

body and encourage a sound night's sleep. Always make sure you are warm enough when trying these out, in order to avoid any risk of getting uncomfortably chilled.

Torso Wrap

Use of a torso wrap every two or three days or a minimum of once a week is thought to improve local circulation to the surface of the skin and improve detoxification and elimination of waste, while also unblocking the pores. Cosmetic benefits include improved skin tone and texture, including a diminished tendency to develop the dreaded cellulite! Regular use of hydrotherapy wraps can help balance energy levels and generally boost immune system functioning, encouraging us to throw off acute illnesses rapidly and efficiently.

1. Line a medium-sized, soft bath towel with a fine piece of slightly damp cotton. The piece of cotton material should be the same size as, or slightly smaller than, the towel. The important thing is to ensure that the damp sheet of cotton doesn't extend beyond the edges of the towel.
2. Wrap the towel tightly around your upper body and pin securely in place. Lie down in a warm room and make sure that the temperature of the damp cotton warms up comfortably. Take it off immediately if it begins to feel uncomfortably chilled. If it feels pleasantly warm, keep the wrap on for approximately 20 minutes before removing it.

N.B. Anyone suffering from circulatory problems should seek medical advice before using hydrotherapy techniques.

Foot Wrap

Strange as it may sound, applying hydrotherapy to the feet can have the beneficial effect of making us feel soothed, calm and ready for sleep.
1. Dip a pair of short, natural cotton socks in cold water and wring them out thoroughly. Put them on, quickly pulling on another pair of thoroughly dry, wool socks on top.
2. Get into a cosy bed you should find you drift off soundly to sleep. As always, make sure your surroundings are comfortably warm in order to avoid becoming chilled, which would be counter-productive when attempting to relax!

The benefits of massage are obvious and undeniable as a hands-on technique for encouraging a state of pleasurable relaxation. Many of us may already have experienced the powerful sense of release of physical tension that comes from having a treatment from a trained massage therapist. Apart from anything else, lying on a massage table in a warm room where we know the pressures of life can't reach us in the form of telephone calls or domestic or professional demands can feel pleasurable in the extreme.

Since massage is so instinctive to us (for instance, how many of us tend to reach out and rub a painful hand or foot if we've accidentally hit it, or stroke the back or shoulder of someone who is distressed and in need of comfort?), we can enjoy the benefits of some basic massage techniques at home. This can be in the form of massaging a partner, friend or family member, or learning some simple self-massage techniques.

If time is short and a full body massage is going to feel a burden rather than a pleasure, don't think that you have to miss out entirely on the benefits of this type of treatment. Instead, limit yourself to working on the areas where most of us tend to hold maximum tension, such as the neck, shoulder, face and head. By letting go of tight, clenched muscles in these specific areas you are likely to feel much more prepared for a sound night's sleep, and will reap the benefits of drifting into a refreshing rest without a struggle.

Simple Massage Techniques

Here are some general guidelines to experiment with. Always bear in mind that you should follow your own instincts, concentrating on some strokes more than others if they feel instinctively relaxing and pleasurable. The pressure that is used should ideally be firm enough to encourage tight and tense muscles to relax, but not so hard that it feels painful or unpleasant.

Make sure that you set up a natural rhythm with whatever strokes you are using, so that your hands keep in almost constant contact with the skin. The best way of avoiding an unpleasant pulling or dragging sensation is to use a light-textured massage oil. Ideas for relaxing, sleep-inducing aromatherapy massage blends can be found in Chapter Eight.

Before beginning a massage, make sure that the surrounding temperature is warm, and that the lighting is pleasantly dimmed rather than bright or harsh. You may choose to have a favourite piece of music playing gently in the background.

It's a good idea to start with the hands, as many of us may keep a lot of tension in our palms, backs of the hands and fingers.

- To begin, warm a little massage oil in the palms of your hands (never apply cold oil directly to the skin!).
- Knead the palm of your right hand with the ball of the thumb of the left. Use firm, circular movements that move outwards in a spiralling motion, until the whole of the right palm feels relaxed.
- Turn your right hand over and repeat the massage action on the back of the hand. Finish off the back of your right hand by making feathery, long stroking movements from the fingers to the wrist.
- Move on to the base of the right thumb, making small, circular movements all the way up, still using the pressure of the ball of your left thumb while supporting your right thumb with your left index finger. Move along each finger on your right hand in this way until the whole hand feels supple and relaxed.
- Repeat the process on your left hand.

You are now ready to move on to your head, neck and shoulders. Starting with the scalp is a good idea, since many of us may overlook the fact that the muscles of the scalp can be a primary seat of tension. This can have the undesirable effect of triggering or aggravating tension in the facial muscles and the jaw.

- Rest the three middle fingers of each hand at the front centre of your hairline.
- Making firm circular movements, move in a direct line along the scalp down the back of your head to the hairline at the back.
- Move back to the front, working your way outwards gradually until the whole scalp is covered.
- Finish off by using the whole of both hands, kneading your scalp rhythmically and gently.

This gives your scalp muscles a much-needed workout, releasing tension and stimulating the blood supply, which benefits the hair follicles.

Massaging Your Face and Head
Starting with both index fingers resting in the middle of your fore-

head where it meets the front of the hairline, make small, circular movements, moving constantly in an outward direction until you reach the temples.

- Move back to your original position at a slightly lower level. Continue until the whole of your forehead has been covered.
- Place your two index fingers at the inner edge of your eyebrows. Making rhythmical pressing movements, move your fingers in a circular fashion tracing around the eye orbit until you reach the point you started from.
- Taking the index and middle fingers of both hands, start from either side of your nose and move across your cheekbones in an outward direction, making small pressing and releasing movements.
- Place both thumbs and the balls of your index fingers just beneath the centre point of your chin. Steadily and slowly move up towards the jawbone area (called the TMJ) using small pinching movements.
- With the palm of each hand, move from your collarbone up your neck, using gentle, rhythmical movements and working from one side to the other until the whole area of your neck has been covered. Ideally, one hand should follow the other in a continuous movement.

Your Chest and Shoulders

Now it's time to work on the front of your chest, where you may be holding an enormous amount of tension without realising it.

- Put two fingers on your collarbone in the central area just beneath the base of your neck. Use the same press-and-release movements described above, moving in an outward direction towards your shoulders.
- Using the three middle fingers of your right hand, make firm, circular movements that cover the areas of tension in the triangular-shaped muscle (called the trapezius) attached to your left shoulder blade.
- Move in a steady outward direction from the spine towards the edge of the shoulder. Spend as long on the side you start with as you need until you feel the area is relaxed and unknotted. Then attend to the other side.

As a final treat, move to the feet. For an especially luxurious feeling, take a little time to prepare your feet for massage by using an exfoliating cream or gel. Many of us forget that our feet take an inordinate amount of punishment each day, only paying attention to them once problems have arisen that cause pain or discomfort. Always remember that relaxed, well-cared-for feet will make us move more freely and, as a result, will make us feel much more relaxed. Concentrate on dry areas with an exfoliator, using firm circular movements: using a preparation that includes peppermint oil can feel especially cooling and reviving to hot, tired, swollen feet.

Moving across the sole using firm, circular movements, spend as much time on the underside of your foot as feels necessary, only moving on to the upper side of the foot when the sole feels thoroughly relaxed and supple.

- Using the fleshy pads of your thumbs, work in circular movements, covering the area from the toes up to the ankle.

The Importance of Regular Exercise

Most of us must be aware by now of the general benefits that come from exercising regularly. Achieving a healthy body shape, stimulating energy levels, enhancing flexibility and improving stamina are all acknowledged improvements associated with taking regular physical exercise.

From the perspective of this book, however, there are very specific advantages of getting physically fit when it comes to the quality and regularity of the sleep we enjoy. These important benefits are linked to the known stress-relieving aspects of appropriate exercise. By providing you with a vital ally against the negative symptoms of excessive stress (these can include any of the following: recurrent tension headaches, muscle tension, fatigue, digestive problems, anxiety, mood swings and/or interrupted or poor sleep patterns), you should find that regular, appropriate physical movement makes you feel more relaxed as well as generally fitter.

On the other hand, the potential variety of exercise regimes to choose from can be confusing. As a result, you may end up feeling at a loss as to where to start.

It's very important to gain a basic understanding of what each system of exercise has to offer so that you can make an informed choice. What follows cannot be an exhaustive run-down of all of the exercise possibilities, but aims to provide a brief sketch of some of the most appropriate methods of exercise available, so you can gain a general idea of the areas of physical movement you may want to explore further.

Safety First

Before considering taking up any form of exercise, anyone who has been a confirmed couch potato should have a quick check at the GP's surgery to make sure that all is well before starting any new fitness regime. Most gyms will provide a physical assessment of this kind on request, but for other forms of exercise (especially anything you're considering taking up unsupervised) it's always a good idea to get checked out first. Obviously this becomes an even more pressing priority if you're having conventional treatment for heart and circulatory problems (including high blood pressure or angina) or if you suffer from any joint and/or muscle pain, stiffness or injury.

Yoga

This is one of my personal favourites, since the benefits that come as a result of yoga practice are so impressively wide. More balanced energy levels, an enhanced sense of mental and emotional relaxation, staggering improvements in flexibility, a leaner body and an awareness of how our breathing patterns are affected by feeling tense and stressed are all acknowledged bonuses that come from becoming adept at yoga.

Yoga provides a refreshing foil to the hyper-competitive aspects of some systems of exercise. In yoga practice we are in competition with no one, and need only to concentrate on our own progress and development. Executing the postures should never feel painful or uncomfortable, since you should always work in harmony with your body's own capabilities. As a result, any risk of injury should be eliminated, since yoga is such a gentle discipline, encouraging optimum levels of harmony between the mind, emotions and body. Don't be misled, on the other hand, into thinking that yoga is a soft option. When practised correctly it is an extremely challenging system of physical movement that can help you build up a formidable amount of physical strength and stamina, while at the same time encouraging the major muscle groups to stretch and lengthen. As a result, you should find that you become more flexible than you ever thought possible.

Since you can choose postures that have either a calming or a stimulating effect, yoga is an immensely flexible tool that you can use in any way you wish. Stimulating yoga routines (such as the Sun Salutation cycle of postures) are best done at the start of the day, while more relaxing postures (including a specific relaxation session which concentrates on diaphragmatic breathing from the abdomen) are best enjoyed in the evening.

Since you need to be doing the postures as accurately as possible in order to derive maximum benefit from them, beginners should initially always attend a yoga class in order to have supervised tuition. Information about qualified teachers may be obtained from the British Wheel of Yoga (see the Useful Addresses chapter).

Aerobic Exercise
Regular aerobic activity that conditions our hearts, lungs and peripheral circulatory system is a well-known ally in protecting us against heart disease. Of course there are also important benefits that come in the shape of greater physical stamina, higher energy levels, a more positive outlook and a more efficient metabolic rate.

In addition, regular aerobic exercise can be an important tool in helping reduce tendencies to develop stress-related symptoms, including poor or disturbed sleep patterns. This is due to the way in which being under unrelieved emotional and mental pressure for too long triggers what is known as the 'fight or flight' stress response.
In other words, too much stress sets off a series of chemical reactions in the body, preparing it for physical action (such as running away from the source of danger or confronting and fighting it). This finely tuned biochemical response involves the secretion of stress hormones including adrenaline which ensure that the heart rate is increased, additional blood is pumped to muscles in order to prepare them for flight, and circulation is drawn away from organs such as the stomach that are not required if we need to fight or run away (this is why we can often feel queasy when tense and stressed).

This is all very helpful when we can take physical action to deal with the stressor, but the fight-or-flight mechanism can lead to health hazards when it's being activated in inappropriate situations.

In other words, if we feel stressed because we're presented with a fierce, man-eating tiger that's chasing us, a bit of help from the fight-or-flight response is likely to come in very handy. But if this same bio-chemical reaction is being set off whenever we're faced with an unreasonable boss shouting at us, receiving an unexpectedly high phone bill or getting drawn into an argument with our kids, it's clear we're going to be in for problems. The most common symptoms that arise from this build-up of mental, emotional and physical stress include high blood pressure, digestive problems, tension headaches, migraines, anxiety and poor-quality, unrefreshing sleep.

This is where aerobic exercise can play an important stress-reducing role, since it allows us to burn off excess adrenaline. By engaging in regular aerobic activity that challenges your heart and lungs within healthy parameters, you should find that you deal with the sources of stress in your life more effectively. This is partly due to the secretion of feel-good chemicals (called endorphins) that are known to be raised as a result of regular aerobic activity, and also down to the fact that you are likely to feel generally physically fitter and more relaxed. This, in turn, should have a noticeably positive impact on your sleep patterns.

To make the most of these positive effects of aerobic activity, it's very important to choose the optimum time of day to exercise, or you may find that it becomes counter-productive. Always avoid exercising too late at night, as it will then be unlikely that you'll be able to switch off afterwards. Early morning is always a good time to choose, since it sets you up well for the day ahead. Alternatively, midday or early evening may suit you better, depending on your individual body clock and temperament.

Most important of all, always make sure that whatever sort of activity you choose is one that you find enjoyable or absorbing, or you can be sure it will fall by the wayside very quickly. After all, who is likely to keep doing something that they feel is boring or unenjoyable? Make your choice from as imaginative a selection as you can in order to match your own individual needs. Appropriate aerobic activities may include any of the following: cycling, swimming, treadmill training, trampolining, rowing, running, 'power' walking or dancing.

Always use common sense when setting about a programme of aerobic fitness: make sure you take it easy at first (5 to 10 minutes of aerobic activity to start with), building up steadily and slowly as your general fitness level increases.

Try this simple test in order to make sure you are working at an optimum aerobic level: if you can maintain a conversation while exercising, you are likely to be working at an aerobic level. On the other hand, if you find you have moved beyond slight breathlessness and are gasping for breath, you are likely to have moved into an anaerobic state, thought to be counter-productive in fitness terms

T'ai Chi

This increasingly popular form of exercise and relaxation combined (sometimes referred to as 'meditation in movement') has a well-established history. Originally developed in China approximately 1,000 years ago as a form of martial art, t'ai chi has come to be regarded as a system with an impressive potential to harmonise mind, emotions and body. When practised regularly with professional guidance, this system of movement can stimulate an enhanced state of calm while improving muscle tone and balancing energy levels.

Although the flowing movements look entirely different when they are performed, t'ai chi does have some striking similarities with yoga. The emphasis on breathing deeply and rhythmically while executing precise movements is an obvious area of common ground, while an improved flow of energy through the body, enhanced muscular relaxation, increased mobility of joints, improved posture and enhanced muscle tone and strength are thought to be potential benefits that come from both systems of movement. Those who would like to improve their physical co-ordination or general mental, emotional and physical balance may benefit especially from learning t'ai chi.

As with other forms of exercise that incorporate postures or movements which must be executed as precisely as possible in order to enjoy the potential benefits (such as yoga or Pilates), a beginner should attend a t'ai chi class regularly in order to learn how to do the basic movements as correctly as possible.

Those of us who suffer from anxious breathing patterns (breathing rapidly and in a shallow way, using only the upper chest) may benefit particularly from regular t'ai chi practice. Once you become aware of how large a part your breathing can play in positively or negatively influencing your state of mind and emotions, you are empowered to change your responses in future. Just feeling more in control at times when you might otherwise experience a sense of powerlessness or helplessness can do a great deal to boost your self-esteem and general sense of being able to cope.

Pilates

Pilates has become immensely popular as a system of exercise over the last decade or so. Originally developed as a specialised physiotherapeutic form of movement by Joseph Pilates in the 1920s, Pilates has gone on to be enjoyed by those who want an exercise system that helps reduce the insidious effects of negative stress on the mind, emotions and body while at the same time giving them access to a fitness programme that helps promote a leaner and longer body shape through improved posture.

The Pilates approach concentrates on doing multiple repetitions of small, controlled movements that isolate and work on specific muscle groups. A basic point of core stability (extending roughly from the bottom of the ribs to the top of the hip bones) is established while executing the Pilates movements, so that the torso remains stable and in a position of optimum alignment throughout. As with yoga, some exercises are done in a standing position, while others are done lying down on an exercise mat. In some studios, specialised equipment may be used to maximise the benefit of each exercise.

Since such precision is needed in order to benefit from Pilates as a system of movement, it comes as no surprise that newcomers to the technique should always learn from a trained teacher. Classes should be small enough to allow for individual assessment of each class member by the teacher. Once the objective of each exercise becomes familiar, it may be helpful to back up class work by using one of the Pilates videos available. However, don't be tempted to use one of these as a starting point, since results may be disappointing if the exercises aren't being performed precisely.

Chapter Five

Nutrition and Sleep

You'd really need to have been living on a desert island for the past decade or so to have remained unaware of the general impact nutrition can have on your state of health and well-being. After all, whenever we open a newspaper or turn on the TV we're constantly being given advice on the basic dietary ingredients that can protect us against heart disease, osteoporosis, digestive problems such as irritable bowel syndrome and other stress-related problems such as migraines.

On the other hand, although in many ways we've never been as well-informed about the impact of what we eat or drink on our health, many of us still fall into common nutritional pitfalls that can aggravate specific health problems. Nowhere is this more true than with regard to stress-related problems such as poor sleep patterns, since there are specific foods and drinks that can contribute to our having a less-than-perfect night's rest.

In addition, eating patterns can also add to specific sleep problems, since having too full or too empty a stomach can prevent our sleeping well. Both of these areas what we eat and when we eat are the subject of this chapter.

Sleep-promoting Foods and Drinks

You may not be in the habit of assessing the relaxing, sleep-promoting potential of the foods and drinks you take, but if you suffer from well-established sleep problems it may be high time to consider this often neglected area of your lifestyle. You may have a fairly accurate idea of the foods and drinks that can contribute to sensations of wakefulness and alertness (these will be examined in detail below), but you may know less about the foods and drinks that can help you relax and unwind when you need to most.

The general principles of a relaxing, energy-balancing diet fall happily within the boundaries of advice that the majority of nutritionists have been giving for the past couple of decades. A diet which is essentially high in unrefined carbohydrates (products or grains that are 'whole' as opposed to refined and white), frequent helpings of beans and pulses, small amounts of protein, plenty of water, with liberal portions of fresh fruit and vegetables and the full spectrum of essential fatty acids in the form of small amounts of cold-pressed virgin olive or sunflower oil, should give you the nutritional fuel you need to feel energised and powered up during the day and healthily relaxed and ready for sleep when it's time for bed.

Having a very light, easily digested late-night snack can help those of us who find that we feel wakeful and restless if we have an empty, rumbling stomach:

- Always choose foods that have sedative properties, such as lettuce, avocado, banana or peanut butter (the latter should obviously be avoided by anyone who has or suspects they have a nut allergy). Any of these can form the filling of a wholemeal sandwich, and they are all rich sources of tryptophan, thought to help promote restful sleep while also having mood-balancing properties.

- If there is no problem with any sensitivity or allergy to citrus fruit (this can sometimes take the form of a skin reaction such as an aggravation of eczema or psoriasis), oranges or mandarins can be a useful late-night snack. This is due to their bromine content, which acts as a sedative, helping to induce a state of mental and physical relaxation.

- Provided you don't suffer from excess mucus production (which can contribute to problems with sinus congestion or coughing at night), a cold or warm glass of milk can help you drift off to sleep. If the milk is warm, adding a dash of honey and cinnamon can enhance the flavour. The extra honey may also help guard against blood sugar levels dropping too rapidly at night, which this can contribute to night sweats.

- Other late-night warm drinks that have a soothing, sleep-inducing effect include herbal infusions that are made from camomile flowers or a blend of several herbs known to relax mind and body. These are likely to come in handy sachets or tea bags that do away with the need for a strainer. Always experiment with several blends until you find a flavour that appeals to your taste buds –

after all, who's likely to feel soothed and calmed if they're gritting their teeth in response to the taste of the infusion they're drinking?

Whether or not you feel the need of a late-night snack to ensure a good night's sleep, you should take a careful look at what you're eating and drinking throughout the day.

- Make sure to include items in your daily diet that are good sources of vitamin B complex.

This group of water-soluble vitamins which includes thiamin, riboflavin, niacin, folate and B12 – plays an important role in supporting the healthy functioning of the nervous system. As a result, when you are getting a healthy, balanced intake of these essential nutrients, you should find that you are less subject to stress-related symptoms such as sleep problems, anxiety and depression.

- Sources of vitamin B complex include: whole-grain products, soya, yeast extract, poultry, fish, nuts, seeds, green leafy vegetables and (small amounts of) red meat.

Your choice of what to eat for dinner is particularly important, and should ideally consist of a healthy portion of carbohydrate (such as brown rice, pasta or potatoes) combined with beans or pulses, a small amount of fish or organic white meat, free-range eggs, or a very small amount of cheese that is naturally fairly low in fat (such as Edam). Always have a large salad to accompany your dinner, as salads are easy to digest and supply important essential nutrients such as antioxidants.

Sleep-inducing Patterns of Eating

The timing and size of your meals can play as important a part in ensuring a good night's rest as the ingredients that are used. As a general rule, common-sense guidelines should always be followed where possible. These include eating dinner at least a couple of hours before retiring: if dinner is eaten much earlier, avoid the potential disturbance of hunger pangs in the early hours by having a very light snack of the kind outlined above.

- In order to keep energy levels as stable as possible during the day (so that you aren't tempted, for example, to have a mid-afternoon nap), make a point of having a plentiful portion of slow-release carbohydrates at breakfast. Avoid the common, crucial mistake of skipping this important start to the day. Combine carbs with fresh fruit that contains fructose (a fruit sugar that is released into our systems more slowly than refined table sugar).

- The same pattern of eating should be observed at lunch, where the complex carbohydrates can be obtained from wholemeal bread or pasta. Be sparing with protein foods, since only a small portion is needed to stimulate the secretion of dopamine (a precursor of adrenaline) which can give us that extra bit of energy we need to help us keep the pace throughout a busy afternoon.
- Avoid indulging in any of the stimulating foods and drinks listed below, particularly at night.

It helps to bear in mind that people can vary, according to our individual sensitivities to certain sleep-disturbing items. Some of us, for example, may find that we need to avoid caffeine from the early afternoon onwards, while others may find that just a cup or two of strong coffee mid-morning can be enough to cause problems in getting to sleep at night.

Foods and Drinks to Avoid

If you want to give yourself the best chance of unwinding at night, it makes sense to try to cut down or give up many of these sleep-hampering substances, as well as introducing those items that have a sleep-inducing effect. As with so many aspects of a healthy lifestyle, what you are essentially trying to establish here is an optimum state of balance, where the basic quality of what you eat and drink on a daily basis is supportive of high-quality health.

Caffeine
Most of us are likely to be aware of the fact that the caffeine present in coffee, strong tea and some fizzy drinks can cause jitteriness, palpitations and wakefulness at night. You may also be aware that additional stress-related symptoms such as migraines, tension headaches, indigestion and urinary tract problems can also be aggravated by too

much caffeine taken on a frequent or routine basis.

What you may not be as aware of is the wide range of foods and drinks that contain caffeine. Any of the following can provide you with surprising helpings of caffeine: chocolate (and that includes chocolate-flavoured cakes, biscuits and ice-creams), over-the-counter drugs (where the caffeine is included as a way of combating the drowsiness that may be caused by other ingredients), prescription medications such as thyroid-balancing drugs, contraceptives, beta-blockers (for the treatment of high blood pressure), combination formulas designed to relieve cold symptoms, or drugs designed to ease headaches. If you are in doubt, always check with your pharmacist.

The following caffeine - content table gives you a quick run-down of the approximate amount of caffeine present in various substances:

Item Approximate	Caffeine Content
1 cup brewed coffee	100 milligrams (mg)
1 cup standard black tea	20–90 mg (depending on the blend and length of brewing time)
1 cup decaffeinated coffee	46 mg
1 cup green tea	40 mg
1 cup instant coffee	70 mg
1 cup chocolate drink	45 mg
1 can cola drink	45 mg
1 can diet cola drink	45 mg
1 tablet caffeinated pain-reliever	45 mg
1 tablet caffeinated cold remedy	37 mg

Alcohol

Alcohol has a rather contradictory effect on our bodies, depending on how much we drink and how often. As a result, many of us may be confused as to whether a stiff drink helps or hinders us when it comes to relaxing and having a good night's sleep.

Generally speaking, an occasional tipple (no more than half a glass of wine or a very small measure of whisky) taken early in the evening with food may have a slightly relaxing effect. It's important to avoid taking even small amounts of alcohol on an empty stomach, however, since alcohol is absorbed much faster into the bloodstream if the extra buffer of food isn't present in the stomach.

Women may also find that they react more strongly to alcohol pre-menstrually or at the time of the menopause, with small amounts having a more marked effect than they would at other times.

Any more alcohol than the amounts mentioned above can have a positively counter-productive effect on your sleep patterns. You are likely to find that you fall asleep quickly, only to wake from an unnaturally deep or fitful sleep with a need to pass water. If you really have had too much to drink, you are also going to find that you have an unpleasantly dry mouth due to the dehydrating effect that alcohol has on the system.

Since alcohol has powerful mood-enhancing qualities, it's also important to bear in mind that those who suffer from anxiety and/or depression may find that their symptoms get more intense after they have had a few drinks. If you are taking medication for either of these conditions, you will most probably already have been advised that alcohol won't mix well with them, and as a result is best avoided. On the other hand, if you aren't taking medication that makes alcohol unsuitable, you may think that a drink or two will help if you are feeling tense or low. Think twice before reaching for the bottle, and opt instead for some of the healthier options discussed above your sleep quality is likely to reap the benefits!

Food Additives
Evidence suggests that sugar and salt can also contribute to a poor, unsatisfying sleep pattern when taken in regular and/or generous quantities.

Salt flavourings such as the ubiquitous monosodium glutamate included in many take-away meals and fast foods appear to be responsible for neurological stimulation. This can result in wakefulness and hyperactivity of mind and body. The latter can be a particularly obvious problem in children, who may show obvious sensitivities and negative reactions to a range of artificial flavourings, colourings and appearance-enhancers.

Foods and drinks that contain a large helping of sugar can also lead to problems with hyperactivity, wakefulness and/or restlessness. Other ingredients to watch out for if hyperactivity and poor sleep pattern are problems include the artificial sweetener aspartame and the food colouring tartrazine.

Sleep-inhibiting Patterns of Eating

- Always avoid having a rich, large or heavy meal just before retiring, regardless of how healthy the ingredients are.

Although the satisfying sensation of having a full stomach can sometimes incline us towards falling off to sleep in double-quick time, digestive problems are sure to raise their head within a few hours' time. This is due to the way that a heavy meal requires very efficient digestive action in order to break down the stomach contents, so that they can move on to the gut. As mentioned in the previous chapters, when we fall into a deep phase of sleep all of our major organs (including the stomach and the rest of the digestive tract) work at a slower, rested pace. While this has a generally beneficial effect by giving these hard-working organs a much-needed rest, if we have a stomach full of food (especially in the case of high-fat foods, since these take more effort to be broken down by the action of stomach acids) the almost inevitable result is likely to be indigestion, heartburn or an unpleasant sensation of queasiness that will most probably wake us from our sleep.

- Don't drink too much before going to bed.
Although it's basic common sense, many of us may forget that any liquid we take in before we retire for the night is going to have to make its way out again (and most probably sooner rather than later!). Whether we are going to have to get up several times during the night in order to pass water or not is dependent on a number of factors, some of which relate to our individual anatomy and age, while others will be determined by the properties of the liquid we've drunk.

For instance, liquids such as tea and coffee are poor choices as late-night drinks, not just because of their caffeine content but also because they have strong diuretic properties which encourage us to eliminate fluid. As a result, after a cup or two of coffee at dinner, we are almost certainly going to have to get up during the night to pass proportionally more fluid than we've drunk in the cups of coffee. The same effect can also happen in response to certain herbal infusions, especially those that are renowned for their fluid-eliminating properties, such as dandelion tea.

Although generally drinking up to 2 litres of water daily is certainly to be recommended, it does make sense to avoid drinking any amount immediately before going to bed, unless we are blessed with an unusually accommodating, generous bladder!

The one exception to this general rule applies if you know you have over-indulged in alcohol, and want to guard against the dehydration that will occur by the time you wake if you don't replace your fluid reserves pretty promptly.

- Try to avoid leaving large gaps between meals or snacks during the day.

Having something small like a piece of fruit, whole-wheat cracker or slice of wholemeal bread every couple of hours or so helps guard against feeling ravenous at night. By having small portions of healthy snacks fairly regularly, you are also encouraging your blood sugar levels to stay as stable as possible. This helps protect against feeling sleepy during the day, with the resulting benefit that you are less likely to reach for that extra burst of energy from a caffeinated drink at night.

Chapter Six

Medicated Sleep: What GPs Have to Offer

Although alternative and complementary medicines have increased significantly in popularity and general use (witness the number of articles that appear regularly in newspapers and glossy magazines, as well as the large expanse of shelf space allotted to over-the-counter complementary medicines in most pharmacies), the majority of us will still usually consult our GP as our first port of call when illness strikes. Sleep problems are no exception to this rule, since established or severe insomnia that's stopping us from leading a fulfilling and creative life on a day-to-day basis can make us feel anxious and panicky. As a result, we're likely to go to our GP in order to try to get the problem sorted out as quickly as possible.

Consulting Your GP for Help

The first obvious question you're likely to be asked when you consult your GP for help with poor-quality sleep is how much stress you're having to deal with on a daily basis. Related questions will explore whether you're suffering from anxiety and/or depression, since both of these conditions tend almost certainly to trigger problems with sleep patterns.

If neither stress, anxiety nor depression seems to be at the root of sleep problems, a perceptive GP will ask questions that relate to lifestyle factors. These questions will most likely focus on your alcohol, tobacco and caffeine consumption, as well as any current conventional medication you are taking. The latter is important, since some orthodox medicines contain caffeine to counteract the drowsiness that can be triggered by other ingredients of the medication. A perfect example of this sort of combination formula may be found in painkillers that combine paracetamol and codeine, with a dose of caffeine being included in order to try to avoid excessive sleepiness caused by the codeine. Taking medication of this kind on a regular basis for the management of back pain or recurrent headaches, for example, can interfere with your sleep without you realising it. This may be especially the case if you're in the habit of taking a dose before bed in order to discourage the pain from coming on during the night.

Some GPs may also enquire whether you find it difficult to switch off and relax, and are likely to explore practical issues such as patterns of work. Clearly those who work variable shifts or who work late into the night, expecting to be able to fall asleep as soon as their heads hit the pillow, are likely to have an uphill struggle on their hands to gain a sound night's rest.

If none of these issues applies, then it will be the task of the GP to investigate if problems with sleep are associated with another, underlying condition. Possibilities might include any of the following: unbalanced thyroid gland functioning (this may take the form of being either over- or underactive), the menopause, pre-menstrual syndrome, asthma or diabetes. Some of these will need to be confirmed by a relevant test (in many cases this may involve nothing more invasive than a blood sample being taken and sent off for analysis).

On the basis of the information that's obtained as a result of this sort of medical interview, it will be the task of the GP to diagnose and treat the problem as best he or she can.

Possible Treatment Options

If the presence of an underlying condition is revealed (such as an over-active thyroid or early menopause), it's likely that treatment will be directed at dealing with the diagnosed condition. Very often, sleep pattern and sleep quality will respond positively as the underlying condition is dealt with.

However, sleep disturbance can be a problem in its own right without being a complication of another health disorder. If this appears to be the case for a patient whom the GP suspects is generally highly stressed, some general advice should be given with regard to the need to take on board relaxation techniques and regular exercise, in addition to pointing out dietary factors that can aggravate sleep problems (such as too much caffeine and/or alcohol being taken on a regular basis).

If relationship problems are also raising overall negative stress levels, some GPs may advise a course of counselling sessions in order to help work through points of conflict. In addition, if a diagnosis of anxiety or depression is reached (especially if it appears that either condition has emerged in response to a short-term trauma), there is a strong likelihood that a course of treatment with antidepressants may be seen as appropriate. More established cases of anxiety and depression may also require additional help from a psychiatrist or psychotherapist, in order to provide maximum support.

Conventional Sleeping Pills: The Pros and Cons

Generally speaking, sleeping tablets are not a popular first choice when a GP is attempting to help a patient with severe or established problems sleeping. This is mainly due to the acknowledged problems with dependence associated with this type of medication, which can occur unacceptably quickly (often within a few weeks of use).

Additional drawbacks include a lessened degree of effectiveness within a relatively short time frame (also often just a few weeks), coupled with a tendency to feel groggy and drowsy on waking. Although the drowsy feeling has a tendency to lift during the course of the day, these tablets are not suitable for anyone who needs to have extremely quick mental and physical reactions. This would apply to anyone whose job involves using machinery or driving on a regular basis.

Sometimes very short-term use of sleeping tablets is justified on the basis that this may be enough to break a negative cycle of wakefulness, especially if there has been an obvious, specific trigger that's set up temporary sleeping problems. A good example of this sort of situation would include acute anticipatory anxiety that descends before an important examination, or the sort of disturbed sleep pattern that can set in after the shock of bereavement. However, many GPs are wary of trying to manage long-term sleep problems with repeated courses of sleeping pills. In general, it's acknowledged that success is much more likely to be forthcoming if the underlying trigger of disturbed sleep is dealt with, rather than relying on merely suppressing the symptoms.

Benzodiazepines

The main concerns about possible psychological and physical dependence are associated with the use of a group of drugs called benzodiazepines. Long-term use of any of these drugs appears to bring with it a significant risk of becoming addicted. In addition, drug-induced sleep involves a different quality of rest, since the drugs are known to work by temporarily chemically depressing brain function. As a result, when we first take sleeping tablets, cycles of REM and deep sleep are greatly reduced. Coming suddenly off sleeping pills after many years of use may also cause problems if this reduction isn't managed carefully and systematically. Common adverse effects of sleeping tablet withdrawal include restlessness, anxiety and wakefulness: symptoms that can be so unpleasant and disruptive that we're tempted just to go back to taking the pills again.

There are newer formulas of sleeping pills that are similar in effect to benzodiazepines. Although these have a similar effect on nerve cells to benzodiazepines, they don't appear to affect our sleep pattern in the same way. As a result, there appear to be fewer problems reported with hangover-type symptoms the morning after. However, we still don't fully know what level of dependence may arise from taking this type of medication, and certain side-effects are already known to arise in some patients. These can include mood swings including aggressive behaviour, and dizziness and poor co-ordination. However, these symptoms are thought to be most noticeable in patients who have a prior history of problems with dependence on benzodiazepines.

Antihistamines
Sometimes GPs will favour prescribing antihistamines, especially if problems with sleep pattern are associated with the presence of allergies. They may also be prescribed for children who have severe problems with wakefulness during the night. Side-effects are pretty varied, and may include any of the following: diminished appetite, drowsiness on waking, dizziness, poor co-ordination, nausea, dry mouth and blurred vision.

Antidepressants
Antidepressants with sedative-type effects can also be prescribed in low dosage where sleep problems have become severe or established. These include the well-established forms of tricyclic drugs, usually taken before retiring to bed at night. Although they are not thought to be associated with as many problems regarding dependence as benzodiazepines, these drugs may also have their disadvan-

tages. These can include a feeling of being hungover on waking and side-effects such as dry mouth, blurred vision, urinary problems and lowered libido.

Patients may be prescribed one of the newer forms of antidepressant if their sleep problems have been sparked off by clinical depression. In such a situation, once their depressive symptoms respond to treatment, the sleep problems also fade into the background. Possible drug options in a situation like this include the SSRI antidepressants.

Other Conventional Medicines

Thankfully, the days are gone when GPs prescribed barbiturates in order to help patients who can't sleep well. Highly addictive in nature, these drugs proved to be hazardous to the point of causing fatalities if mixed with alcohol or taken in overdose.

Occasionally, one of the chloral drugs might still be prescribed. Generally thought to be less effective than benzodiazepines, one of the problems associated with this type of drug is a tendency to escalate the dosage in order to achieve the effect that was forthcoming at the beginning of use.

Can Alternative Medical Support Work Alongside Conventional Drugs?

Generally speaking, most of the complementary therapies mentioned within the scope of this book can be used side by side with conventional medication such as sleeping tablets or antidepressants. In fact, some of them, such as homoeopathy, can provide you with a very important avenue of support if you are cutting down on your conventional medication with the advice, guidance and monitoring of your GP. This vital help from complementary medical sources can provide you with a dual benefit, since the positive physiological effect on both mind and body provided by these therapies can help regulate and improve sleep pattern.

In addition, having an extra avenue of practical support can give you a positive form of psychological comfort in the knowledge that you don't have to go completely 'cold turkey'. This is especially valuable to anyone who, despite their best efforts, knows that they've developed a psychological dependence on their sleeping pills and is very nervous of coming off them.

The one area where you need to take extra care is with regard to taking herbal preparations, since some of them can either interfere with the effective action of conventional medication or can sometimes have the effect of magnifying the effect of whatever orthodox drugs are being prescribed. This is obviously an issue of concern where sedative effects are involved, since exaggerating these can be extremely unwise, or in some cases dangerous.

St John's Wort and Kava Kava

Two current examples of this problem are St John's Wort (Hypericum), which is an extremely effective herbal treatment for the relief of symptoms of mild to moderate depression, and Kava Kava, which has been used with success in relieving the symptoms of anxiety and sleeplessness. The main problem with combining St John's Wort with conventional antidepressants is that the herbal alternative can interfere with the medicinal action of the orthodox antidepressant.

Kava Kava should not be combined with any other sedative medication, since it can enhance the sedative effect to an undesirable level. It may also have been responsible for a small number of cases of liver damage in Europe. As a result, it should be avoided by anyone with a history of liver problems; everyone else should seek an opinion from a qualified medical herbalist before embarking on self-prescribing.

There are other groups of specific drugs that may also be adversely affected by taking St John's Wort, so it's generally best always to check with your pharmacist, GP or alternative health practitioner if you are in any doubt about the compatibility between any herbal and conventional drugs that you may be taking. As a basic rule: when in doubt, always ask!

An Alternative Approach

Some of us may choose a non-conventional medical approach as our first port of call if we begin to experience sleep problems. Exploring an alternative approach of this kind can be a sensible course of action, especially if you want to try to solve sleep problems without resorting to sleeping pills in the first instance. The next chapter takes a look at the alternative and complementary medicines that can help.

Chapter Seven

The Alternative Medical Approach

Alternative and complementary medicines have an enormous amount to offer those who want to investigate a gentle but effective form of treatment that can help restore a healthy sleep pattern. This can be an especially appropriate avenue of medical support for those who are wary of the undesirable side-effects that can be associated with conventional drug treatments such as sleeping pills.

Many people may think that the idea of using alternative or complementary therapies is all very well and good, but surely, since they have a reputation for working in a natural and gentle way, they must take a very long time to achieve any effective result. This mistaken assumption can also be unwittingly encouraged by the marketing imagery used to sell conventional medications. Very often these advertisements rely on aggressive images of high-tech, targeted delivery of relief to the problem area, combined with a high-speed response.

The reality of treatment with alternative or complementary therapies is, however, often a delightful surprise to patients, since positive results can often be unexpectedly swift in coming. Ironically, when patients react particularly well to alternative measures, they often comment on how much faster and more decisively they have obtained relief from their symptoms than they have in the past with conventional medication. The key is finding the most appropriate form of alternative treatment for each individual patient. Once this has been done, a patient and his or her family and friends can end up being converted to alternative or complementary medical treatment for life, often using it as their first port of call whenever illness sets in.

The Whole Picture

For many alternative therapists, sleep patterns and sleep quality are vitally important indicators of general health. This is partly due to the

way that sleep can be adversely affected by so many medical conditions. As you have seen in the previous chapters, anxiety, depression,
tension headaches, migraines, thyroid disorders, ME, pre-menstrual
syndrome and the menopause are just some of the disorders which
can have a major impact on the quality of the sleep we enjoy on a
regular basis. In many cases, sleep disruption is one of the very first
symptoms to emerge as ill health is developing.

By the same token, a lack of sleep, or poor-quality sleep that continues unabated, can leave us vulnerable to so many additional problems. These may include any of the following: reduced immune
system functioning, mood swings and a severe and persistent feeling
of mental, emotional and physical fatigue.

This is why alternative therapists will often pay a great deal of attention to evaluating each patient's sleep quality and pattern, regardless
of the condition that has brought the patient in for treatment. Each
therapist will have a different approach according to his or her own
discipline (for instance, a practitioner of traditional Chinese medicine will spend a great deal of time examining the pulse and the tongue, while a homoeopath is more likely to want to explore the mental
and emotional state of the patient), but there is a strand of central
importance that runs through all alternative therapies that fall into
the general classification of *holistic* approaches to healing.

This strand consists of treating each patient as an individual, and
taking time to explore how he or she is experiencing the illness on
more than a purely physical level. In contrast to the average GP,
who is likely to give patients approximately eight minutes of consultation, an alternative practitioner will often spend an hour to an hour
and a half on the initial appointment. This time is spent exploring
each patient's medical history, nutritional status, ability to relax,
energy levels and state of mental and emotional balance.

As you can imagine, if sleep problems have emerged as a relatively
new phenomenon say as a result of a traumatic experience a sensitive alternative practitioner will have the time and space to explore
the event that has triggered the sleep problem. Although the event
cannot be erased from the patient's consciousness, some alternative
and complementary therapies are very well placed to support a
patient in coming to terms with and moving on from feelings of
repressed grief, shock or anger.

More long-term sleep problems which are being aggravated by certain lifestyle aspects, such as an absence of effective stress-management techniques, a sedentary pattern of working or a general lack of physical exercise, or unhealthy eating and drinking patterns, are also likely to come to light during an in-depth exploratory interview with an alternative practitioner. This information may emerge either in response to perceptively asked, sensitively put questions, or as a result of clues that emerge from physical examination. Either way, the patient is given an invaluable therapeutic space within which to explore lifestyle issues that may be aggravating his or her sleep problems. The possibility of healthy change that is opened up by this sort of professional exchange can lay the bedrock for improvement, so that whatever alternative or complementary medication is prescribed will have the maximum opportunity to work well.

Certain systems of alternative medicine, such as Ayurveda and homoeopathy, can also have a very important role to play in addressing sleep problems that have an identifiable pattern each night. In other words, if a patient has a tendency to wake on the dot at 2 o'clock each morning, this will provide an important clue to the choice of homoeopathic remedy selected for that person. Ayurvedic medicine, on the other hand, lays particular emphasis on the patterns of ebbing and flowing energy levels in each individual person. By identifying imbalances in the flow of vitality in each patient, an Ayurvedic practitioner is in a position to give practical advice with regard to restoring an optimum energy balance. When a harmonious and balanced flow of energy in the body is established by effective treatment, sleep patterns also benefit. (For more information on the Ayurvedic approach to individual body types, see page 91 in Chapter Eight.)

What Alternative Medicine Has to Offer

While alternative and complementary medicines can't work miracles, anyone battling with a persistent or severe sleep problem should certainly consider seeking help from this valuable and appropriate source.

It's important to bear in mind that alternative therapies can be applied alongside conventional medication. In other words, you shouldn't feel under pressure to give up conventional medicine if you want to reap the benefits of an alternative medical approach. This is especially important in cases where drugs such as oral or inhaled steroids (commonly used to treat asthma or arthritis), beta-blockers or ACE inhibitors (usually prescribed for high blood pressure), or lithium (prescribed to control symptoms of bipolar disorder or very severe symptoms of anxiety and depression) have been taken for an extended period of time. Since these drugs should not be withdrawn abruptly due to the possibility of a negative rebound effect, any alternative therapist who offers treatment must be prepared to treat patients in a truly complementary way, prescribing what they offer side-by-side with conventional treatment. In this way it is to be hoped that, as the overall condition of the patient slowly and steadily improves, a responsibly monitored reduction of conventional medication supervised by a GP or hospital consultant may become a possibility further down the line.

This has particular relevance for those who experience sleep problems as part and parcel of another condition such as anxiety, depression, ME or menopausal symptoms. Once you begin to respond positively to alternative treatment, you should find that you develop not only a very real sense of well-being but also increased energy levels and much-improved sleep on a regular basis. When treatment has worked especially well, this should embrace both the quality and duration of your sleep.

Therapies such as Western medical herbalism, homoeopathy, traditional Chinese herbalism and aromatherapy all have the undeniable benefit of providing you with an extra source of practical support if you're trying to phase out or cut down on sleeping tablets or tranquillisers.

This effectively side-steps one of the well-known, toughest aspects of reducing habit-forming conventional drugs such as sleeping tablets: the unpleasant psychological dependence that is a common experience of anyone who has taken sleeping pills for an extended period of time. Many patients treated with these drugs have experienced a basic dilemma, knowing rationally that the sleeping tablets they take each night have long ago stopped having any positive medicinal effect, but feeling they need to continue taking them because there is just a chance that the ritual of taking them may be what gets them off to sleep.

Having an alternative, non-habit forming medicine that can be taken without running the risk of feeling 'hungover' and groggy in the morning can also be an invaluable avenue of psychological and practical support. It also helps discourage the risk of taking ever stronger doses of sedative medication to achieve the same effect.

It's important to bear in mind that since most alternative and complementary approaches to healing are attempting to improve the quality of health of each patient right across the board, they provide a very streamlined approach to treatment. This is likely to come as a refreshing change to those who are used to being sent to a different specialist for every distinct health problem the neurologist for unexplained migraines or headaches, the gynaecologist for menstrual problems, the endocrinologist for suspected diabetes, etc. Since any or all of these problems can arise in one patient in the course of his or her life, with each disorder needing treatment with a different drug (plus possibly extra drugs to deal with side-effects brought on by the various medications!) it's very easy for the dosages taken on a daily basis to escalate to undesirable levels.

Many alternative and complementary therapists, on the other hand, will strive to get a patient's whole system back into balance with a minimum of therapeutic stimulation. As a result, you may be surprised to find that just one course of homoeopathic tablets or herbal liquids, selected especially for your individual constitution and range of symptoms, will be all that is required. The simplicity of this approach is likely to be particularly appealing to anyone who doesn't like the idea of taking a large amount or lots of different medications.

It also helps to know that alternative medical treatment is an especially appropriate option to consider for those who have more recently developed sleep problems within the context of generally good health. When an alternative practitioner is presented with a patient who has had the minimum amount of conventional medical intervention, and who in addition appears to have a generally robust constitution, he or she can expect to see a rapid, clear, positive response to treatment. This is partly due to the way those of us who have resilient constitutions tend to have healthy mental, emotional and physical energy reserves to work with. It's also a huge bonus for an alternative or complementary practitioner to work with cases where the original symptoms are clear-cut, rather than having their work cut out in trying to evaluate which symptoms are due to side-effects from whatever conventional medication is being taken, and which symptoms stem from the original, underlying health problem.

Self-help vs Professional Treatment

When to Seek Qualified Alternative Medical Help
For self-prescribing to have the best chance of working efficiently, safely and speedily, you need to work within firm, practical boundaries so that there is no risk that you will get out of your depth. If any of the following occurs, it would suggest that you would benefit from consulting a trained practitioner rather than soldiering on alone.

- Symptoms that appear to be becoming more severe rather than showing signs of definite improvement within a reasonable period of time (a sensible period of time for this evaluation would be approximately three to four weeks)
- Signs that suggest the situation was initially improving in response to self-help, followed by a relapse after a few weeks although still taking the chosen alternative or complementary medicine
- If your sleep problems emerge in association with another, chronic condition such as anxiety, depression, ME or fibromyalgia

As a general rule of thumb, the most suitable conditions that can be treated successfully with alternative and/or complementary prescribing at home are generally those that fall into the acute category. These problems are easy to spot, since they tend to have a predictable life-span, and will often clear up of their own accord provided enough time and support is available in the form of positive lifestyle adjustments. Good examples of acute conditions include stomach upsets, colds, uncomplicated bouts of flu (without a background history of bronchitis, asthma or sinusitis), or sleeplessness that has developed in response to a specific trigger such as a period of intense stress, bereavement or short-term worries.

Treatment of chronic conditions, on the other hand, should generally be placed in the hands of a trained practitioner for the best chance of success. Chronic problems tend by their nature to be well-established conditions that do not clear up under their own steam, but tend to be subject to repeated flare-ups over time. Since the case-management of chronic conditions can be a complex business that requires a great deal of experience on the part of the practitioner before a successful resolution can be reached, this is a classic situation where home prescribers can drift out of their depth. Excellent examples of chronic conditions are asthma, eczema, irritable bowel syndrome, hay fever, depression, recurrent or very severe anxiety, and osteo- or rheumatoid arthritis.

Sleep problems that arise in conjunction with pre-menstrual syndrome or the menopause (the latter may intensify problems in the sleep department through the frequency of night sweats) also respond best to professional alternative treatment. This is due to the way that the treatment selected will be aimed not just at improving sleep quality, but at the more ambitious task of getting your entire system into as optimum a state of balance as possible. As a result, when treatment is successful, specific symptoms associated with hormone imbalances (hot flushes or erratic and/or painful periods, for example) will be rectified along with other general symptoms such as erratic energy levels, mood swings and sleep disturbances.

Even if the pointers listed above suggest that it would be helpful to seek professional alternative or complementary advice and treatment, this does not mean that you can't also benefit from the positive lifestyle changes outlined in this book. General self-help of this kind can only be a positive help, supporting whatever therapies a conventional medical practitioner or alternative or complementary therapist suggests. Any positive adjustments you make to your lifestyle can only give whatever treatment you are receiving a head start and a helping hand along the way.

Chapter Eight

Aromatherapy, Herbal and Homoeopathic Self-help

This chapter is designed to give you a quick tour of some of the practical alternative and complementary measures you can draw on in order to improve the pattern or quality of your sleep. It must be stressed that this is very much a whistle-stop approach rather than an in-depth evaluation of each therapy. If you discover that you're motivated to find out more about any of the therapies mentioned, the list of books in the Recommended Reading chapter will point you in the right direction.

Before we take a look at the over-the-counter products that you might consider if you want to get to grips with a bout of disturbed sleep, you need to grasp some of the basic background to these therapies, so that you know a little of what is involved with each approach. This is worth doing because, although there are certain common themes running through each therapy mentioned, there are also essential differences in practical application that give each healing system its own individual perspective and approach with regard to treatment.

Although Ayurvedic and traditional Chinese medicine are not appropriate for self-help measures, a little of the background to these therapies is given, since each has something important to offer in the treatment of sleep problems. These types of therapies are, however, best received from a trained practitioner for the best chance of successful treatment.

Aromatherapy

Aromatherapy has become an immensely popular complementary therapy over recent years. The reasons for this aren't hard to guess, since the application of essential oils in the form of massage, inhalation or in the bath is more often than not a highly pleasurable experience. In addition, it is very much a practical, 'hands on' therapy that you can approach with less trepidation than some of the more esoteric therapies which can seem much more complex and inaccessible.

The history of the use of aromatic oils for healing purposes goes back a considerable way, with evidence existing to show that perfumed oils were used for embalming as far back as ancient Egyptian times. The ancient Greeks also seem to have been sensitive to the mood-enhancing qualities of floral fragrances, and appear to have made use of perfumes, aromatic baths and healing ointments in health-promoting regimes.

Aromatherapy has a particularly established basis in Europe, with essential oils being used – diluted in a suitable carrier oil and in combination with massage – as a way of easing a number of health problems. Aromatherapists are trained to treat patients who suffer from a wide range of chronic conditions such as stress-related problems (including tension headaches, migraines, mood swings and digestive disorders) and sleep problems, as well as chronic skin disorders such as eczema and psoriasis.

The training an aromatherapist receives is quite comprehensive in nature, demanding that the trainee therapist grasps a full and detailed understanding of the healing properties of different essential oils, in addition to learning about basic anatomy and physiology.

A consultation with an aromatherapist should involve going through a basic case history where you will be required to explore your experience of health on an emotional, mental and physical level. Once this information has been assimilated and analysed, it's the job of the aromatherapist to select the appropriate blend of essential oils that will most closely suit your individual needs. Whatever blend is selected is usually applied to the skin in the form of an aromatherapy massage, or it may be inhaled. While some aromatherapists elsewhere in Europe prescribe essential oils that can be taken by mouth, this is something that is not advocated in Britain by practitioners. It is certainly something that should *never* be attempted by the self-prescriber at home.

Aromatherapy falls into the category of a holistic therapy, which seeks to stimulate an improved state of overall health in each patient rather than aiming at the piecemeal treatment of isolated symptoms. As a result of this comprehensive approach, at an initial consultation some time is likely to be spent exploring lifestyle issues which are acknowledged to have a positive or negative effect on emotional, mental and physical health.

This exploration may include practical advice on diet, exercise, relaxation techniques and effective stress-management measures. As seen in previous chapters of this book, these issues are well worth exploring due to the significant impact they can have on sleep quality.

If we take the following simple example, you can begin to appreciate how lifestyle factors can form a sort of jigsaw: when the pieces are in place, a positive health picture emerges; when they're not, you get a negative picture that steadily undermines your experience of health.

If a patient consults an aromatherapist in an attempt to relieve chronic muscle tension that's leading to constant aches, pains and fatigue, the treatment outcomes may proceed like this:

- Because the patient responds well to having a relaxing blend of essential oils applied to his tight, previously untouched muscles, he may also start using a relaxing blend of essential oils in a soothing bath each night.
- As a result, he is likely to sleep more soundly and comfortably, which should have the desirable effect of stimulating healthier, steadier levels of energy and stamina.
- Once his fatigue is less intense, there is a good chance that taking the trouble to eat and drink more wisely will become a reality rather than remaining nothing more than a good intention.
- As more progress is made and a sense of increased relaxation becomes a reality, there's a strong possibility that the patient will want to build on this positive spiral by learning about systems of movement such as yoga or t'ai chi, which help to stretch and relax tense muscles.

And so the positive spiral is encouraged to continue …

Self-help for Sleep Problems

Generally speaking, as with any of the other holistic therapies outlined below, those who suffer from well-established or extremely severe sleep problems should consult a professional practitioner if they want to derive maximum benefit from this therapy and allow for the best chance of success.

However, if you have begun to suffer from mild symptoms of disturbed sleep that clearly relate to a perceptible trigger (too many late nights, temporary escalation of stress or an acute bout of illness such as a heavy cold or dose of flu), you may be able to get things back on track again in double-quick time by trying any of the following self-help measures.

Any of the following essential oils may be used diluted in a carrier or base oil (this provides a vehicle for safely diluting essential oils, and can come in the form of almond, jojoba, olive, safflower or sunflower oil) for a relaxing aromatherapy self-massage or massage from your partner or a friend. Alternatively, a few drops may be dropped onto your pillow to be inhaled overnight, or a sparing amount (no more than a maximum of 5 drops) can be added to a soothing, warm bath before retiring, or vaporised in a custom-made vaporiser in the bedroom:

- Mandarin
- Camomile (to be avoided by those who are pregnant or who have sensitive skin)
- Hops (to be avoided by those who have sensitive skin, are depressed, or are suffering from fatigue)
- Lavender
- Ylang ylang
- Frankincense (to be avoided in pregnancy)

Always remember to dilute a very sparing amount of essential oil in a carrier oil. Never apply aromatherapy oils directly to the surface of the skin. For most favourable results, add 2 or 3 drops of your selected essential oils to every 5 ml of carrier oil.

When adding essential oils to the bath water, always add a small amount (no more than 5 drops) to the warm bath water, making sure that the taps have been switched off. This is important in order to allow the perfumed oil to float on top of the warm water so that it can release its perfume slowly; dropping the oil in as the hot tap is running, will encourage the oil too quickly.

Ayurvedic Medicine

Ayurvedic medicine is a holistic system of healing that has been used for generations in Asia and is becoming more popular in the West.

This is partly due to the work of high-profile practitioners such as Deepak Chopra, who have interpreted Ayurvedic principles and made them accessible and relevant to a Western context with its particular pressures, stresses and problems.

From the Ayurvedic perspective, each patient's individual constitution is influenced by three basic *doshas* (these can be understood as vital energies or elements). These are called *Vata* (wind energy), *Pitta* (fire energy) and *Kapha* (earth energy).

The three doshas are thought to be present in some proportion in all of us, with one being dominant. When *Vata* energy is dominant, staying power can be a problem due to erratic mental, emotional and physical energy reserves, a strong tendency to be easily distracted, flightiness, insecurity, anxiety and high levels of vitality which can be dramatically and quickly exhausted.

Those who have dominant *Pitta* characteristics are likely to be passionate, energetic, enthusiastic, quick-witted, alert and ambitious, with a tendency to rapid irritability and lack of patience.

Kapha types are more given to listlessness, sleepiness, tranquillity, patience and contentedness, with a general tendency to lack of emotional, mental and physical stamina, and lack of flexibility.

When the three doshas are in balance, we should experience optimum health on all levels. However, life so often intervenes and too much stress, eating or drinking unwisely, financial problems, bereavement, pregnancy, looking after a newborn baby, retirement or coping with a difficult menopause can all be responsible for setting off an imbalance that results in symptoms of lacklustre health and vitality. And, as has been seen, poor sleep patterns can be among the leading indicators that all is not well in the health department.

Since Ayurvedic practitioners aim to treat the whole person, gently stimulating the mind, emotions, body and energy levels back to good health, this can have huge benefits for those who are struggling with chronic or severe sleep problems.

Self-help
Ayurvedic medicine is not really a therapy that can be applied successfully within a self-help context, but if this approach to healing sounds interesting or attractive, it's worth considering a course of Ayurvedic treatment from a qualified practitioner.

Although Ayurvedic medicine is much more readily available in India, physicians trained in this holistic medical system also work in the United States and the United Kingdom, where treatment can be obtained from Indian-trained practitioners or from conventional doctors who have pursued additional training in Ayurvedic medicine.

During a consultation, Ayurvedic physicians make use of their skills of observation as well as gathering as much information as possible about your current and past medical history. In doing so, questions are likely to be asked about your personal and professional life, eating and drinking habits, sleep patterns and experience of energy. A physical examination is likely to involve reading your pulse and checking the appearance of your tongue, eyes, skin, hair and nails.

Once this information has been gathered, it's the task of the physician to decide on the most appropriate course of therapeutic action. This could involve the prescription of medicines made from herbal, mineral or vegetable sources, advice on dietary changes, use of breathing techniques, fasting regimes, steam baths, massage, oil treatments, exercise, relaxation or detox regimes.

It's worth bearing in mind that you don't have to wait for symptoms of ill health to emerge before you seek help from an Ayurvedic physician, because this is an excellent therapeutic choice to make if you want to pursue the idea of genuinely preventative treatment.

Herbal Medicine

Magazine articles and news snippets commonly refer to herbal medicine as if it were just one thing, often overlooking the fact that there are two distinct branches of herbal medicine, each of which has a rich, extended and fascinating history. These different but related approaches to herbal treatment are of Western medical herbalism and traditional Chinese medicine (which includes treatment using herbal preparations).

Chinese Herbal Medicine

Consulting a practitioner of traditional Chinese medicine is a very different experience from popping into the average GP's surgery for an appointment. The first thing that's likely to strike you is the practitioner's extremely detailed examination of your tongue and pulses. Pulse-reading gives the practitioner a major clue to the eventual diagnosis that's reached, since certain qualities of the pulse's strength, rapidity and regularity – examined in a way that goes far beyond the attention paid to the pulse by a GP working in Western conventional medicine are all thought to have a bearing on the overall health of the patient.

Interestingly, the tone and strength of the voice of the patient may also be noted, since this can be a useful clue to the patient's state of mind. Because traditional Chinese practitioners apply a holistic approach to treatment, any additional clues that can be pointers to the patient's state of mind are considered of particular value.

Once all the relevant information has been gathered and assimilated, it's the job of the therapist to select a prescription of herbs that will suit each individual patient. This prescription can come in a variety of different forms, including liquid tinctures, powders and pills. In some cases, a mixture of dried herbs may be given to the patient. In such cases these are given with the intention that the herbs are to be simmered in a pan of water and the resulting liquid to be drained off and drunk. This is called a *decoction*. Sometimes pills or tinctures may be chosen in preference to this method, due to the often strong taste of decoctions.

In addition to the use of herbal preparations, traditional Chinese practitioners may also use acupuncture to stimulate the mind, body and emotions gently towards an enhanced state of balance. Although traditional Chinese medicine has attracted a great deal of positive attention with regard to its successful treatment of chronic skin disorders such as eczema and psoriasis, its potential benefits are by no means confined to these conditions. Patients can also consider this form of holistic treatment if they are seeking relief from stress-related conditions (including sleep disturbance), asthma, allergies, pre-menstrual syndrome, menopausal problems, migraines, digestive disorders, recurrent minor infections or arthritis.

Western Medical Herbalism
Western medical herbalism has a fascinating, long and established pedigree, with a comprehensive body of practical knowledge that has been built up on a 'hands on' and trial-and-error basis over an impressive number of years.

It can come as a refreshing surprise to realise that conventional medicine relies on a surprisingly large number of drugs derived from plant and herbal sources. However, while these plants and herbs are undoubtedly the starting points for both herbal and conventional drugs, the way in which they are used differs in a significant way.

When conventional drugs are produced, one of the main objectives is to isolate and develop a concentrated, measurable extract of the ingredient in the plant that is regarded as having the active, medicinal effect. Although this approach clearly brings practical advantages (including the ability to work with finely tuned and specifically measurable doses of the pharmacologically active ingredient), there is also a downside to this approach that has become increasingly obvious over the years. This to the side-effects so often linked to using conventional drugs that are based on concentrated extracts of plants.

Western medical herbalists work from a contrasting perspective, maintaining that there are perceptible gains to be made from using the *whole* plant rather than a highly concentrated extract of one component of the basic substance.

One of the major advantages thought to be associated with using whole plants is related to something called the *synergistic* effect. This simply means that using the plant as a whole allows the medicinal effect of any one chemical compound contained within the plant to act as a buffer against the others. Herbalists maintain that this allows for a more balanced, less drastic effect with possibly fewer risks of side-effects.

To give a quick example: the popular conventional drug aspirin was originally obtained from a plant source. Once the pain-relieving effects of the compound acetylsalicylic acid were effectively isolated, the drug aspirin was born. However, this was only partly successful, since although this drug provides us with a very effective source of pain relief, used over an extended period of time it can give rise to problems with stomach irritation and low-grade bleeding.

Western medical herbalists also make use of the same substance but, by utilising the medicinal potential of the whole plant, a much gentler, less toxic effect is produced. This is connected to the way in which the salicylate content of the plant acts as a very effective analgesic and anti-inflammatory, while the tannin and soothing mucilage content yielded by the same plant act as important medicinal buffers, making it less likely that unwelcome digestive side-effects are going to emerge.

When a patient consults a Western medical herbalist, he or she can anticipate a very thorough examination. In the course of such a consultation, extremely detailed information will be gathered about the patient's general, basic levels of health and vitality, as well as an impression of his or her overall diet, lifestyle and stress-management levels. The pulse and blood pressure readings are most likely to be taken, and questions will be asked about any existing medical conditions and conventional drugs that are being taken on a regular basis.

A herbalist may also examine the iris of your eye (a technique known as iridology) as an additional diagnostic tool. By examining the patterns and flecks of the iris, it is believed to be possible to identify weaknesses or problems within specific organs or systems of the body.

Once all of this information has been gathered and assessed by the herbal practitioner, a course of treatment can be embarked upon. More often than not, this will involve a prescription of herbs selected for each patient's specific set of problems, in an attempt to stimulate a healing, balancing response. In some cases, this may involve the prescription of herbs that have specific anti-inflammatory or antibiotic properties, or in others it may be necessary to concentrate on those that have relaxant, tonic or stimulating qualities.

In addition to whichever herbal prescription is selected, you may also be given general advice on adjustments to your lifestyle that will be supportive of better health. This could involve recommendations with regard to exercise or relaxation techniques, combined with dietary improvements.

Self-help
One of the best ways of gaining confidence with using herbal self-help is to start with some simple herbal teas. These are increasingly available in an ever wider range of possibilities ranging from single herbs to more sophisticated blends put together in order to achieve a specific effect (for instance calming, relaxing, invigorating or stimulating).

If sleeplessness has become a nuisance, you would do well to try drinking a cup of a soothing, relaxing herbal tea before retiring. This provides an excellent alternative bedtime drink free of any of the drawbacks of caffeinated beverages. Appropriate choices include any of the following:

- Camomile
- Limeflower
- Valerian

Alternatively, you can make use of the soothing qualities of herbs as topical preparations in the simple forms of infusions that can be used to make a relaxing bath or footbath.

To make a bath-time infusion, add three generous handfuls of your selected herb to a pan of cold water. Leave to stand overnight, then bring to the boil and strain off the liquid and keep it in a screw-top jar with a closely fitting lid. Add this to the bath water and soak. Suitable herbs to choose would include:

- Camomile
- Limeflower
- Lavender
- Passionflower

Alternatively, you can place any of the herbs listed above in a fine muslin bag and suspend it beneath the hot tap as the bath water is running.

If you have a tendency to sensitive skin, it's best to try single herbs at first, just to minimise any temporary itching or irritation. Obviously, if this should occur it's best to avoid that particular herb in future.

For those who feel they hold a lot of tiredness, stress and tension in their feet by the end of a busy day, a herbal footbath can be just what's needed. Just add a strong infusion of camomile tea to a bowl of warm water (if time is tight, just throw in a herbal tea bag or two), soak your feet up to the ankles, sit back, close your eyes and relax.

Although strictly speaking not just a herbal preparation, a few drops of *Avena sativa* tincture taken in a small glass of water just before retiring can be an excellent, non-addictive support in helping you switch off after a stressful day. Made from a combination of herbal ingredients such as valerian, hops, oats and passionflower, it provides an ideal alternative if you have come off conventional sleeping pills and feel a bit lost without some temporary extra help to nod off. Once your sleep pattern becomes more regular and your level of confidence builds with regard to achieving a good night's sleep, you can dispense with the *Avena* sativa.

Alternatively, you may choose to try valerian compound tablets. These are made from herbal ingredients (including hops, valerian and wild lettuce).

Note
If you are already taking conventional drugs of any kind, check with your pharmacist or GP before starting a course of herbal self-help medication. This is worth doing in order to eliminate the possibility of any potentially counter-productive effects. Cautions that apply to this sort of combination of herbal ingredients include not giving herbal tablets to children under the age of 12, and avoiding taking them in pregnancy or when breastfeeding.

Homoeopathic Medicine

Although it has been in existence for over 200 years, general public awareness of homoeopathic medicine has grown considerably over the last decade or so. I've noticed this change in a very personal way: whenever I was asked what I did for a living in the late eighties, it was clear that most people had no clue what a homoeopath was. Now, times have clearly changed, since heads theses days nod enthusiastically in recognition at the mention of homoeopathic treatment.

One of the main reasons for the popularity of the homoeopathic method of healing is its gentle but effective approach, which aims to guide mind, emotions and body in the direction of optimum balance and harmony. When this holistic therapy is effective, it should result in a corresponding improvement in mental and emotional well-being in proportion alongside the treatment of physical symptoms. As a delightful and surprising bonus, many patients discover that their base-line levels of energy and vitality are also restored as a result of successful homoeopathic treatment.

It helps to remember that homoeopathy was developed over two centuries ago as an alternative, gentle system of healing in response to the excesses of conventional medicine. Samuel Hahnemann, the doctor credited with setting the science of homoeopathy in motion, was originally trained as a conventional physician. However, as he saw the effect of conventional treatment on his patients, he became increasingly alienated, feeling that he was doing more harm than good by his efforts.

In response to this disillusionment with the orthodox medical approach of his day, Hahnemann began to conduct a series of controlled experiments using increasingly diluted medicines in the hope that distressing side-effects would be measurably reduced. The result of these experiments was the development of the theory and practice of homoeopathic medicine, a process that continued over the course of Hahnemann's lengthy and prestigious career as he constantly sought to refine and improve further the treatment available to his patients.

Homoeopathic medicines are quite different to conventional drugs in two important ways. The first relates to their astonishingly dilute nature: they are diluted to a point where it is extremely unlikely that any molecules of the starting substance are left in any given dose. The second is linked to the significant concept of using *similars* rather than opposites when selecting substances that are intended to have a medicinal effect. As we are already aware, most orthodox drugs work by counteracting whatever bodily reactions seem to be causing a problem. So it seems logical that conventional doctors prescribe anti-inflammatories when attempting to calm inflammation and pain, or laxatives for stubborn constipation, or antibiotics for bacterial infections.

Homoeopaths, however, prescribe medicines that have a 'similar' rather than opposing *effect*. In other words, substances are used that would actually trigger symptoms in a healthy person if given in a non-diluted form for long enough. These same substances work therapeutically when prescribed for a sick person in the form of a minute, energised dose. Provided the patient's symptoms closely match those that are known to be produced by the substance that's been given, this proves an effective form of treatment.

When this match is as accurate as it can be, the homoeopathic medicine appears to act as a catalyst, 'kick-starting' the self-healing potential of the body. However, if a totally inappropriate medicine is chosen (i.e. one that bears little or no resemblance to the characteristic symptoms of the patient), nothing of positive effect is likely to happen.

The central importance of matching the individual symptoms of the patient to the most appropriate homoeopathic remedy is the rationale behind the lengthy and detailed nature of any initial consultation with a homoeopath. This will usually take anything up to an hour and a half, and during the course of the consultation the practitioner is likely to ask you a surprisingly wide variety and range of questions. These are basically aimed at giving the homoeopath a general impression of how you experience ill health in your own specific, individual way. Possible areas that are likely to be explored include your ability to deal with stress, your general levels of energy and well-being, the quality of your sleep, your resistance to infection and your overall ability to focus and concentrate, in addition to the specific health problem that brought you to the homoeopath's consulting room in the first place.

In addition, details of your family's medical history will need to be taken, in order to explore the possibility of patterns of illness being handed down through the generations.

Once all of this information has been gathered and assimilated, it's the task of the practitioner to choose the homoeopathic remedy that will match your symptoms most accurately. This process is called *case analysis*, and may be done using textbooks called a *repertory* (listings of symptoms) and *Materia Medica* (listings of remedies and their effects). However, it's increasingly the case that practitioners will use computer programmes designed with the intention of making case analysis and choosing the most appropriate homoeopathic remedy much faster and more efficient.

Most patients are extremely pleased to discover that a successful reaction to homoeopathic treatment doesn't involve taking homoeopathic remedies on a long-term or permanent basis. Once treatment has stimulated a positive response that is then sustained for an established period of time, homoeopathic support can be appropriately phased out. This is due to the way that homoeopathic medicines act as catalysts, giving your body's own self-regulating and self-curative potential a kick-start or a boost. Once this has been set decisively in motion, no additional homoeopathic support is likely to be needed, unless a relapse occurs further down the line.

The time taken for this positive effect to emerge can vary significantly from patient to patient: some may need no more than a few months' treatment, while more complex, severe or well-established cases may take years of treatment depending on the patient's overall

vitality, age, amount of conventional treatment received and suscept-
ibility to homoeopathic medical support. As always, what matters
most is the unique requirement of each individual patient, a principle
that lies at the very heart of the homoeopathic approach to healing.

Self-help
Where sleep problems are concerned, homoeopathic self-prescribing
can be an invaluable help in giving you access to an alternative avenue
of support if you want to avoid using conventional sleeping pills. Alternatively, if you want to come off these tablets and feel you need something to act as a therapeutic buffer in order to make the transition more
gentle and successful, homoeopathic medicines can also be extremely helpful.

As stated in earlier chapters, if sleep problems are well established or
severe (especially if you are taking conventional drugs), you really
need to consult a homoeopathic practitioner for the best chance of
success. However, short-lived sleep problems that make their appearance as a result of an identifiable trigger (too many late nights, temporary escalating stress levels or emotional upset) can respond very
effectively to a short course of a well-selected homoeopathic remedy.

When homoeopathy works well for sleeping problems, it appears to
support the body in switching off mentally and physically. Of course,
this effect is further enhanced if you make an effort to cut down on
foods and drinks that may be making it harder for you to achieve this
effect.

Most important of all, bear in mind that whichever remedy is chosen
must match your own symptoms as closely as possible for improvement to follow. Sadly, a totally unsuitable remedy taken over a couple
of doses will do absolutely nothing helpful for you in the sleep stakes.

As far as dosage goes, the most commonly available doses from
pharmacies and health food stores are the 6c potency. Occasionally,
30c potencies may be found (these have a stronger effect than a 6c
dose). For treating mild symptoms of recent onset, the selected
remedy should be fine given in a 6c potency three times daily for two
or three days. If symptoms have rectified themselves by the third day,
be sure to stop taking the remedy at this point, since no more needs to
be taken unless a relapse should occur at a later point.

For symptoms that seem only marginally improved by a 6c potency,
or that keep relapsing after a short time, it may be worth trying the

same homoeopathic remedy in a 30c potency, taken twice daily for two to three days.

Always bear in mind that over-the-counter homoeopathic remedies are not intended to be taken on an extended or daily basis. If you find you need to take them frequently in order to maintain a positive effect, it's time to consult a trained practitioner who will be able to provide you with more deep-seated, effective treatment.

The following are all commonly indicated homoeopathic remedies for short-term sleep disturbance:

Aconite
This remedy can help significantly with short-term sleep problems that set in after a traumatic, upsetting experience. Common symptoms include restlessness, anxiety, palpitations and panic, all of which are worse when in bed at night.

Arsenicum album
This can help sleep disturbance that results from someone pushing themselves too hard mentally and physically. Consequently, it can often be needed by anyone who sets very high standards for themselves, and who refuses to cut themselves essential emotional slack at times of high stress and pressure. There's a tendency to fall asleep quite easily but to wake feeling anxious at around 2 a.m. There may be associated queasiness and/or diarrhoea when under pressure.

Nux vomica
Candidates for burn-out are almost certain to need this remedy at some point. Classic symptoms that suggest this remedy is appropriate include a marked tendency to rely on stimulants to keep the pace. So, a common pattern is likely to include drinking gallons of strong coffee in an effort to keep the pace, while using cigarettes and alcohol in a desperate attempt to relax and unwind. Not surprisingly, additional symptoms include headaches, irritability and digestive problems such as persistent constipation and/or indigestion.

Lachesis
This remedy can be extremely helpful for 'night owls' who go through phases of bursts of creativity late at night, with a resulting problem in switching off in the early hours of the morning. When this sort of

cycle sets in, waking feels awful because you are not fully rested or refreshed. Those who do well with this remedy are likely to find that they are subject to a brief.

Ignatia

Sleep problems that date from a time of unresolved grief can be helped greatly by this remedy. Characteristic symptoms include severe difficulty in falling off to sleep, with lots of yawning and possible tics and twitches as the body and mind resist relaxation. As a result of poor sleep patterns, mood swings are likely to be marked during the day, often shifting quite rapidly from feeling positive and upbeat to sudden bouts of tearfulness. Unpleasant dreams or recurrent nightmares can also benefit from this remedy if they date from the shock of bereavement or emotional loss.

Rhus tox

If sleep is elusive because of muscular aches and pains at night, this is a remedy worth considering. Characteristic symptoms include maddening physical restlessness at night which triggers a state of persistent wakefulness. It's also good in cases where an episode of joint or muscle pain may have been triggered by a snap of cold, damp weather. Once awake, feelings of depression or despondency move in during the early hours of the morning.

Bryonia

If you have difficulty dropping off to sleep in the early hours of the morning as a result of thoughts of work crowding in, you may do well with this remedy. Since persistent thoughts of professional or domestic concerns interfere with drifting off to sleep, once you can get some sleep these anxieties may be worked out through dreams, and you'll feel better during the day as well.

Combination Formulas

If you find it hard to match your individual symptoms to any of the above homoeopathic remedies, don't give up. There is another homoeopathic approach that may help. This comes in the form of a custom-made combination formula of homoeopathic remedies selected with a view to easing the symptoms of disturbed or fitful sleep. The taking of more than one homoeopathic remedy at a time runs contrary to the classical school of homoeopathic prescribing (an approach that is very popular in the UK), but falls in line with patterns of homoeopathic prescribing found in the rest of Europe and parts of the United States. Although these formulas are certainly worth trying, if they don't work, don't automatically regard this as evidence that homoeopathy doesn't work or that you may be resistant to treatment. At this stage it would be worth considering treatment from a homoeopathic practitioner, especially if your problems are very severe or well established.

Obtaining Good-quality Alternative and Complementary Medicines

Thankfully, the days are gone when it was an uphill struggle to find a basic range of herbal or homoeopathic medicines, since distribution and availability was limited to specialist outlets. These days anyone should be able to find most of the remedies mentioned in this chapter at a local high street pharmacy.

If you can't find what you're looking for, however, your next stop should be your local health food shop. Alternatively, many specialist outlets such as homoeopathic pharmacies provide a mail order service. See the Useful Addresses chapter for suppliers of herbal, homoeopathic and aromatherapy products.

Hints that the Self-prescriber May Be Getting Out of Their Depth

Should any of the following occur, it's always a good idea to consult a professional alternative and complementary medical practitioner:
- an initial improvement isn't holding.
- escalating doses seem to be required.
- additional signs and symptoms appear as this suggests that the situation may be more complicated than a case of simple, short-lived sleep disturbance (symptoms to look out for include loss of appetite, tearfulness for no obvious reason, irritability, poor concentration, feeling uncharacteristically withdrawn, or changes in alcohol consumption).

- no improvement has been forthcoming in response to self-help measures that have continued over a number of weeks.
- Any well-established conditions tend to fall into a category that's often referred to as *chronic* in nature. Since chronic health problems can be extremely complex as well as deep-seated, they are best treated by a professional practitioner rather than by self-help measures alone.

Quick Hints on Coming Off Conventional Sleeping Tablets

Before kicking the sleeping pill habit, take a few weeks to make some helpful lifestyle changes that will be supportive of a successful outcome. Some basic adjustments to consider include cutting down on or cutting out coffee, strong tea, alcohol and fizzy, caffeinated drinks; taking up relaxation techniques (see Chapter Nine; using soothing aromatherapy essential oils creatively; and incorporating some regular exercise into your daily routine.

- If sleeping tablets have been taken for an extended time (months or years) it's always helpful to inform your GP or family physician that your intention is to come off the medication. This gives you the opportunity of receiving specific guidance on how best to reduce medication successfully.
- When choosing a time to come off medication, it's very important to avoid any phases when your stress levels are going to be high or where you may be spending time away from home. Factors such as these are likely to burden you with extra obstacles to success, and you really don't need these at a time when you're attempting to regulate your sleep patterns.
- Some forms of complementary and alternative medicines such as homoeopathic remedies or aromatherapy essential oils can be used side by side with conventional sleeping tablets, but always check with your pharmacist or GP about the suitability of specific herbal medicines. This is very important, since some of these are incompatible with certain conventional drugs, including sleeping tablets.

Never attempt to cut down the dose of your sleeping tablets abruptly or drastically. A much more successful outcome is likely to ensue after slowly and systematically reducing the dose. So, for instance, if you take one tablet each night, it would be sensible to halve this dose for a night and see how you cope (as already mentioned, some complementary therapies can be a useful additional support during this transitional phase). Then go back to the full dose for one night, but reduce the dose to half for the following two nights. This process can be slowly continued, steadily extending the phases when half a dose is taken. If after a month this system is working well, take half a dose on the nights when a normal dose would be taken, and a quarter of a dose on the nights when you've been taking half. After another month, take a quarter of a dose every other night. If all is well, this can be further extended to a quarter of a dose every three nights, four nights, until it becomes once a week, and then stops altogether.

Tedious as this may seem on first consideration, this gentle, progressive regime is well worth making the effort to try, since it's far more likely to yield positive results than the 'short, sharp shock' approach.

Chapter Nine

Stress-reduction Techniques that Promote Sound Sleep

Stress seems to be the buzz word on everyone's lips these days. We all seem to have an opinion on this controversial subject, whether we believe it's one of the greatest blights on 21st-century life, or nod our heads enthusiastically in agreement with those who feel stress is an indulgence reserved only for wimps.

The chances are that the answer lies somewhere in between these two extreme points of view. Although not all stress is negative, it certainly appears to be true that unmanaged, escalating negative stress levels can have an extremely destructive and disruptive effect on the quality of life we enjoy on a day-to-day basis.

Most significantly from the perspective of this book, a lack of effective stress-management techniques can result in a very undesirable knock-on effect with regard to the duration and quality of the sleep we enjoy on a regular basis. The specific reasons for this are briefly explained in the next section.

The Fight-or-flight Response

As mentioned earlier, whenever we're faced with a situation we perceive as stressful, our bodies automatically respond by setting in motion something called the 'fight-or-flight' reaction. The basic function of this process is to support our bodies in taking prompt, decisive physical action in the face of a threat. Any changes that take place in our bodies as a result of the fight-or-flight mechanism are tailored to support us in taking whatever course of action is appropriate for meeting the crisis. This could involve anything from engaging in physical combat to sprinting away from the source of the threat in double-quick time.

In order to provide us with maximum support in taking either course of action, our bodies need to undergo a series of involuntary changes (in other words, changes that are outside the realm of our conscious control). Consequently, blood sugar levels are raised to give us an energy boost, secretion of the two major stress hormones cortisol and adrenaline is increased (which in turn raises blood pressure and makes the heart beat faster), breathing becomes accelerated and shallow, digestive activity is virtually locked down, and muscles are provided with an increased supply of blood in order to give us a better chance of sprinting away from or fighting off the danger.

As you may imagine, while this is extremely helpful in enabling us to respond effectively to a threat that demands physical action, it's much less appropriate if we're needing to deal with a stress factor that can't be run away from or punched in the jaw! As a result, stress-related problems tend to arise if we're faced with an array of subtler pressures that make us feel psychologically stressed but which can't appropriately be dealt with by taking physical action. Good examples of this type of stress include constant pressure to meet unrealistic deadlines at work, financial difficulties, relationship problems that involve lack of or poor communication, or regularly being shouted at unfairly by our boss at work.

If these sorts of situations arise on a regular basis and the fight-or-flight response is being triggered frequently at a low-grade level, it's an unpleasant fact that a host of health problems will begin to emerge.

Since stress hormones such as adrenaline are responsible for making us feel extremely alert and edgy, you can imagine that any excess adrenaline that's not being burnt off by vigorous exercise is eventually going to wreak havoc in the sleep department. Poorly managed high stress levels are also almost certain to contribute to feelings of anxiety, agitation, palpitations, muscle aches and stiffness, and tension headaches none of which is going to help us gain a relaxing night's rest.

Thankfully, there is a practical strategy at your disposal for defusing the negative effect of escalating stress. This invaluable de-stressing tool is known as *the relaxation response*, and the beauty of it is that once you're familiar with what's involved, you can use it at a moment's notice.

The Positive Benefits of the Relaxation Response

In the past it was thought that we could control the voluntary functions of our bodies (such as speaking, running or eating), but that we had no hope of influencing involuntary processes such as fluctuations in blood pressure, rate of heartbeat or body temperature. However, ground-breaking work carried out by writers such as Dr Herbert Benson (author of *The Relaxation Response* and *Beyond the Relaxation Response*) has demonstrated that we can indeed positively influence bodily functions that were previously thought to be beyond any conscious influence.

By studying subjects who are capable of inducing a state of profound relaxation or meditation, it was revealed that it is possible to dramatically lower blood pressure and to regulate respiration, heartbeat, and even body temperature.

This prompted an extraordinary change in our perception of what might be possible through effective relaxation, since it demonstrated that we can exert conscious control over a bodily system that was previously regarded as unreachable (the parasympathetic branch of the nervous system).

Once you are able to bring into play the influence of the parasympathetic nervous system through effective, regular relaxation or meditation techniques, a host of positive developments tend to follow: reduced anxiety, sounder sleep, reduced blood pressure, less of a tendency to be mentally and emotionally volatile, and enhanced powers of concentration.

Various tests run during the experience of deep relaxation confirm the other benefits of being able to control the parasympathetic nervous system: reduced oxygen absorption, slower heart rate and a significant reduction in measurements of blood lactate levels. This last appears to be especially significant, because raised blood lactate levels are thought to be associated with symptoms of increased anxiety. As a result, when we trigger the relaxation response, we appear to move into a profoundly relaxed mode of being that can be confirmed by objective tests and measurements of physical functions.

The possible avenues of deep relaxation available are extremely wide. Depending on your individual taste and temperament, they may include any of the following: autogenic training, biofeedback, transcendental meditation, progressive muscular relaxation or creative visualisation.

In the sections that follow we will explore some of these relaxation techniques, concentrating on those that can be approached from the perspective of self-help. While autogenic training, biofeedback and transcendental meditation are undoubtedly beneficial with regard to inducing a state of effective relaxation, these are best learned with the help of a trained practitioner teacher for the best chance of success.

General Guidelines for Effective Relaxation

- Create a soothing and tranquil space to relax in. Unplug the telephone, dim the lights and choose the quietest room at your disposal. Also tell family members that you aren't under any circumstances to be disturbed for at least half an hour. If it helps, choose a room that has a lockable door like the bathroom (provided, of course, that the floor is comfortable!).
- As body temperature has a surprising tendency to drop during deep relaxation, make sure that you are warmly dressed and that the room is comfortably warm and cosy. However, avoid poorly ventilated surroundings, as they're likely to make you feel drowsy. You might think that if you fall asleep the effect is much the same as deep relaxation, but this is not the case. One of the crucial differences lies in the presence of slow (alpha) brain-waves. Not generally present during sleep, alpha waves are thought to characterise a state of deep relaxation. If you do inadvertently nod off in the course of a relaxation exercise, it's not a disaster, but it may leave you feeling disorientated and groggy rather than refreshed and calm.
- Wear loose and comfortable clothing. If clothing is too tight or restrictive around the neck or waistband, there's a fighting chance that it's going to distract you and, as any of you who are newcomers to relaxation know, it can be quite an uphill struggle to clear your mind of distracting thoughts in the first place!
- You may choose to sit upright during meditation or a relaxation exercise. If this is the case, always use a straight-backed chair that gives adequate support to your spine. Being hunched over has a strongly counter-productive effect on relaxation by instinctively triggering shallow breathing patterns. As you'll discover once you get into the instructions for the simple exercises that follow, full breathing is the key to effective relaxation.
- Most important of all, try to make relaxation a regular part of your daily routine. Don't get stressed out if you miss a day or two (after all, this would rather defeat the object of the exercise!), but do

make a point of resuming your relaxation routine as soon as possible.

- When using relaxation exercises to help induce improved sleep, it can be especially helpful to get into the habit of relaxing just before bed in order to help prepare your mind for sleep. It's probably best to avoid doing any of these exercises once comfortably tucked up in bed, since there's a strong chance that you won't get very far before nodding off! Desirable as this may seem at first glance, you won't gain their maximum benefit in the long term if you're unable to go through the full relaxation routine on a regular basis.

Meditation: How to Set About It

Those who reap the benefits of daily meditation are extremely enthusiastic about the way in which it can help us to deal with a wide range of tension-related health problems. These can include anxiety, poor-quality sleep, high blood pressure, lack of mental focus and mental and physical lethargy.

Put very simply, effective meditation can be regarded as a way of switching off the background noise or 'chatter' that goes on constantly in your mind. When you are uptight or anxious, you may feel as though the volume of these distracting thoughts gets louder, having the undesirable effect of making you even more uptight and unfocused. Once you begin to meditate effectively you'll be giving yourself a vital tool for switching off these random thoughts, with the result that you should feel more relaxed, clear-headed and focused throughout the day.

The techniques used in meditation may sound surprisingly simple: the challenge is most likely to come from applying the discipline of making time and space for regular practice. Ironically, this can seem most difficult at the very times you need them most: in other words, during phases of high stress and pressure.

You can sit upright or lie down when meditating: it's really up to you. Opt for whichever position feels most relaxing and comfortable. Remember that this can vary from day to day, depending on your mood. If choosing to sit, make sure that your spine is well supported and upright, and that your feet feel relaxed and make comfortable contact with the floor. You might find that sitting on the floor in a cross-legged or kneeling position feels comfortable, but always avoid doing this if it results in any discomfort or tension in your knees or back. After all, any signals of pain are just going to make emptying your mind of niggling or distracting thoughts an even bigger challenge.

If lying down, make sure that the surface you're lying on feels draught-free and comfortable. It can be helpful when lying flat to adopt the yoga relaxation posture called 'the Corpse', the name of which pretty much speaks for itself! In this position you should lie flat on your back with your arms relaxed and away from your body at a slight angle and the backs of your hands making gentle contact with the floor. Your fingers may naturally curl inwards towards your palms. Your legs should also be at a slight angle and apart (anything resembling hip-width is fine). Make sure that the small of your back isn't arched but makes comfortable contact with the floor this ensures that you're not putting undue strain on your back muscles.

If you are seated, one method of meditation is to focus on an object such as a flower or candle flame. Focus on the object (always remembering to blink at regular intervals or your eyes will get sore and tired), deliberately putting other thoughts to one side as they flit through your mind (and you can be certain they are going to do this with a vengeance at first).

- Close your eyes and begin to pay attention to your breathing, making a mental note of how deep, rapid or irregular it may be.
- While gently concentrating your gaze on your chosen object, or on an image in your mind's eye if you prefer, slowly bring your attention to the rhythm and speed of your breathing. Without forcing anything, gently regulate your breathing so that it begins to take on a balanced rhythm, with the intake of breath being equal in length to the out-breath.
- It's often helpful to repeat a simple sound to yourself, of no more than a single syllable. You could, for instance, try repeating the word 'one' slowly to yourself while concentrating on your breathing. Don't feel bound by this, but choose any sound that appeals to you as you try to clear your mind of distracting thoughts.
- At first, you may try this for no longer than five minutes, building up the time spent meditating according to the time available to you. Always remember: the most important thing is regularity

rather than time spent during each session. For instance, it's better to spend five minutes meditating every day than half an hour every week.

- Never be tempted to rush at the end of meditation, since your mind and body need time to adjust to regular activity once more. Once you're ready, slowly open your eyes, move your head gently from side to side, stretch your arms and legs, and get up very slowly. If you have been lying down, never sit up abruptly, but turn on to one side, taking time to get used to the change in position before slowly sitting up.

Simple Creative Visualisation Techniques

Visualisation is nothing more complicated than taking a regular, pleasurable mental holiday. All it takes is the ability to call up an image you associate with especially relaxing, positive qualities. When preparing to do this, follow the suggestions given above for a meditation session.

- Once comfortable, focus your attention on your breathing and check that it's steady and rhythmical. Try to clear your mind of any intruding thoughts, and begin to visualise a scene that you find especially beautiful, inspiring, secure and soothing. Don't feel limited to places that you may have visited; you are free to conjure up your own imaginary setting, or one that you may have found especially moving in a photograph, television programme or painting. The essential thing is that this needs to be a place with which you feel you have an instinctive rapport.
- As you mentally enter the scene, begin to immerse yourself in the surroundings. The more detailed you are regarding the setting, the more rewarding your experience is likely to be. Imagine the sights, sounds, aromas and feel of the place. You may choose to 'walk' slowly though this place, discovering fresh aspects of the scene that draw you even deeper into a state of relaxation. Alternatively you may imagine yourself lying down at a chosen spot and luxuriating in the sense of calm that floods over you.
- At this point you may feel you want to draw your guided relaxation session to a close. If so, just follow the suggestions given above for how to do so safely. On the other hand, if you wish to take the

experience of relaxation further, you can move on to some progressive muscular relaxation techniques.

Progressive Muscular Relaxation

- Begin by concentrating on the muscles of your face and scalp.
  Starting at the crown of your head, visualise letting go of any tension that you sense is being held in the muscles of your scalp.
  Move steadily down your forehead and face, paying attention to
  any tight muscles that you encounter on the way. Consciously
  focus on each knot of muscle tension, tensing and releasing each
  group of muscles before moving on.
- Pay particular attention to any sense of tautness that may be lying
  around the area of your jaw. If this feels especially tight, rest the tip
  of your tongue for a second against the back of your top teeth
  while you breathe out gently.
- Move down your body, systematically relaxing any tense muscle
  groups you find on your journey. Common areas where muscle
  tension tends to be held include the neck, throat, shoulders,
  hands and lower back.
- Once you get used to the sensation of progressive relaxation, you
  should experience a delightful sense of calmness and deep
  relaxation. You may feel as though your body has become much
  heavier and is sinking through the floor, or the opposite sensation
  can occur where you feel so light you seem to be floating. These
  are both quite normal reactions to experiencing a state of deep
  relaxation.
- Once you feel all areas of tension have been dealt with, take a
  deep, slow in-breath and imagine you are being filled from the
  crown of your head to the soles of your feet with a sense of profound, positive calm. As you slowly breathe out, visualise any
  traces of tension and negative energy being gently expelled from
  your body.
- You may find this easier if you choose a colour to symbolise the
  sense of calm that floods your body and another that stands for
  the tension that is leaving it. These may change from session to
  session in tune with your mood.
- Bask in this profoundly relaxed state for as long as you wish or

practicalities dictate, but always ensure that you allow plenty of time to emerge slowly and gently from this state of mental and physical tranquillity. After all, having taken so much care to induce a state of relaxation, it would be a shame to diminish the resulting benefits by rushing back too quickly to activity.

Once you are ready, start by slowly bringing your attention back to your surroundings. Initially, make small, gentle movements with your head, shoulders, arms, fingers, legs and toes. Gradually increase the size of the movements until you are naturally making larger flexing and stretching movements. Enjoy a big, cat-like stretch before opening your eyes.

If you have done this session at the end of your day, this is a perfect moment for soaking in an aromatherapy-scented warm bath, having a cup of soothing herbal tea and climbing into bed.

At this point, all that remains to be said is 'sweet dreams'.

Recommended Reading

Deepak Chopra, *Restful Sleep: The Complete Mind-Body Programme for Overcoming Insomnia* (Ebury, 2000)

Dr Chris Idzikowski, *The Insomnia Kit: Everything You Need for a Good Night's Sleep* (Newleaf, 1999)

Leslie Kenton and Susannah Kenton, *Endless Energy for Women on the Move* (Vermillion, 1993)

Sheila Lavery, *The Healing Power of Sleep: How to Achieve Restorative Sleep Naturally* (Gaia, 1997)

Beth MacEoin, *How to Cope Successfully with Anxiety and Depression* (Wellhouse Publishing Ltd, 2001)

Beth MacEoin, *Natural Medicine: A Practical Guide to Family Health* (Bloomsbury 1999)

Beth MacEoin, *The Total De-Stress Plan: A Complete Guide to Working with Positive and Negative Stress* (Carlton Books, 2002)

Michael Van Straten, *The Good Sleep Guide* (Kyle Cathie, 1996)

Bharti Vyas, Beauty Wisdom: *The Secret of Looking and Feeling Fabulous* (Thorsons 1997)

John Wiedman, *Desperately Seeking Snoozin': The Insomnia Cure from Awake to ZZZZZ* (Towering Pines Press Inc, 1999)

Useful Addresses

Aromatherapy Organisations Council
PO Box 19834
London SE25 6WF
Tel/Fax: 020 8251 7912

Ayurvedic Living
PO Box 188
Exeter
Devon EX4 5AB

British Acupuncture Council
Park House
206208 Latimer Road
London W10 6RE
Tel: 020 8964 0333
e-mail: info@acupuncture.org.uk

British Wheel of Yoga
1 Hamilton Place
Boston Road
Sleaford
Lincs NG34 7ES
Tel/Fax: 01529 303233

National Institute of Medical Herbalists
56 Longbrooke Street
Exeter
Devon EX4 8HA
Tel: 01392 420622

The Nutri Centre
The Hale Clinic
7 Park Crescent
London W1N 3HE
Tel: 020 7436 5122

The Society of Homoeopaths
2 Artizan Road
Northampton NN1 4HU
Tel: 01604 621400
website: www.nhsconfed.net/bha

Society for the Promotion of Nutritional Therapy
BCM Box SPNT
London WC1N 3XX
Tel: 01825 872921

T'ai Chi Union of Great Britain
94 Felsham Road
London SW15 1DQ
Tel: 020 8780 1063

Other titles available from

Wellhouse Publishing

HOW TO COPE SUCCESSFULLY WITH

DIVERTICULITIS

Dr Joan McClelland

Diverticulitis is a Cinderella disorder. It is very common, can be dangerous and there are rapidly increasing numbers of sufferers. We stand a more than 50 per cent chance of suffering from diverticulitis before we reach the age of 60. Dr Joan McClelland describes in her easily accessible style the symptoms, different types of diverticulitis, complications and various treatments including alternative and herbal remedies. This book also covers the psychological aspects of diverticulitis and the benefits of exercise and diet.

ISBN: 1-903784-00-X

128pp

HOW TO COPE SUCCESSFULLY WITH

ANXIETY AND DEPRESSION

Beth MacEoin

We live in stressful times and have to cope on a daily basis with a variety of different pressures. These can include financial worries, emotional stresses, bereavement, break-up of relationships and insecurity at work. When feeling well and resilient we are able to cope with a wide range of these stressful situations. It is when we become mentally and emotionally overloaded at a vulnerable time in our lives that we can suffer from symptoms of anxiety or depression. Beth MacEoin describes in her easily accessible style the various symptoms and suggests a wide range of practical measures to provide positive support.

ISBN: 1-903784-03-4

128pp

YOUR LIFESTYLE DIET

Karen Sullivan

A healthy diet is more than just balancing food intake, it involves eating foods that promote rather than endanger health. What are the elements of a healthy balanced diet? How do we identify which are good fats, bad fats and essential fats? What problems can be caused by sugar in our diet? What are the different types of sugars found in our diet and which are healthy? What should we drink and what should we avoid drinking? What essential supplements do we need? The answers to these questions and many more are contained in Your Lifestyle Diet.

ISBN: 1-903784-04-2   128pp

MENOPAUSE

Dr Joan McClelland

The menopause is an event to welcome, a stimulating new chapter in your life. You can say goodbye to period pains, water retention, PMS together with a host of psychological problems including irritability, depression and chronic tension. The menopause is a vantage point from which to take stock, reviewing your earlier life and looking ahead to new interests, deepening relationships and fresh goals. You are entering an important and fascinating time in your life and to get the best out of it you need to work in harmony with nature, this book aims to help you achieve this aim.

ISBN: 1-903784-05-0   128pp

DIABETES

Dr Tom Smith

If there was ever a role model for people with diabetes, insulin-dependent or otherwise, Sir Stephen Redgrave is it. Few people with diabetes aspire to his Olympic gold medal heights but everyone can take heart from the way he put his body through the most rigorous training and still kept good control of his diabetes. The main aim of this book is to achieve a good quality of life despite the health hiccup of diabetes. This book describes all aspects of the healthy lifestyle that every person with diabetes needs to follow, it is positive and optimistic to give people with diabetes a sense that they can shape their own future.

ISBN: 1-903784-02-6

128pp

THYROID PROBLEMS

Dr Tom Smith

The thyroid is not a subject that immediately springs to mind when we chat socially about our health. We marvel how some people have boundless energy while others are always tired and weary. There are nervous, anxious, agitated people who can never sit still. It is easy to assume that people differ in these ways because of their characters or lifestyle but a substantial number have developed these characteristics through no fault of their own. These are the sufferers from thyroid problems. Do Tom Smith describes in his easily accessible style the symptoms, different types of thyroid problems, complications and the various treatments available today.

ISBN: 1-903784-01-8

128pp

HIGH BLOOD PRESSURE

Dr Duncan Dymond

Blood Pressure is not a disease, everyone has a pressure, we need it to keep us upright and alive. Your blood pressure varies depending on your level of physical and mental stress. In this easily accessible book Dr Dymond describes what high blood pressure is, the symptoms, various medications available, side effects and possible complications. The tests and investigations for high blood pressure are explained together with treatments and suggestions for changes to lifestyle and diet.

ISBN: 1-903784-07-7   128pp

PANIC ATTACKS

Karen Sullivan

Panic attacks are a much more common problem than is generally realised an affect a large proportion of the population. They can manifest themselves in many ways including agoraphobia, anticipatory anxiety, separation anxiety, school or work phobia. This book explains what Panic Attacks are, the causes, how panic affects daily life and the associated disorders. Conventional treatments together with their side effects are explained and alternative remedies including acupuncture, homoeopathy, reflexology, massage are covered. Karen Sullivan gives reassuring short term measures to help deal with an attack and, together with other advice, Top Ten Tips to help cope in the longer term.

ISBN: 1-903784-08-5   128pp

IRRITABLE BOWEL SYNDROME

Richard Emerson

Irritable Bowel Syndrome is a complex problem with both physical and psychological symptoms. The aim of this book is to set out clearly and concisely these symptoms and the various treatments now available – conventional, complementary and alternative. Ths should enable sufferers to improve their lifestyle and either cure or manage their Irritable Bowel Syndrome.

ISBN: 1-903784-06-9

128pp

CANDIDA THE DRUG-FREE WAY

Jo Dunbar

Candida is the common name for an overgrowth of yeast organism known as *Candida Albicans*. Candida appears with many seemingly unrelated symptoms – it affects almost every part of the body and has become an umbrella term for any collection of symptoms of no identified cause. Because of the wide range of symptoms and the lack of positive diagnostic tests available, this gap has provided fertile ground for individuals of limited medical training to quickly hop on the band wagon and begin 'diagnosing' Candida for almost any condition or illness.

This book introduces a thorough drug-free treatment program, as well as tips on how to adapt your life-style to treating Candida.

ISBN: 1-903784-11-5

128pp

HOW TO COPE SUCCESSFULLY WITH

COLITIS

Dr Tom Smith

We know a lot about the changes that occur in the bowel of people with colitis and how to return them to normal. It should be only a matter of time before we know *why* these changes happen. Colitis means 'inflammation of the large bowel' (the colon), inflammation takes several forms and doctors have different views from the general public on what constitutes colitis. Most of this book is devoted to ulcerative colitis and Crohn's, with chapters on how to distinguish these inflammatory bowel diseases from irritable bowel, diverticular disease and colon cancer.

ISBN: 1-903784-12-3   128pp

HOW TO COPE SUCCESSFULLY WITH

HIGH CHOLESTEROL

Dr Tom Smith

We are all becoming more aware of high cholesterol problems and often only discover that we are at risk when having a geneneral health check. In this book Dr Tom Smith describes in his easily accessible style the causes of high cholesterol, the associated problems, the complications and the risks involved if your high cholesterol goes untreated. Dr Tom Smith details the treatments available together with possible side effects. He also gives information on diet and lifestyle changes which may be needed to help reduce your cholesterol levels and reduce the risks to your overall health.

ISBN: 1-903784-09-3   128pp

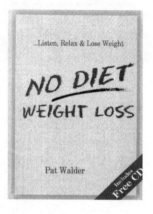

NO DIET WEIGHT LOSS

Pat Walder

- Have you tried of an endless variety of diets?
- Do you find you lose some weight, then put it all back on again - plus a little more?
- Do you envy those people who can eat whatever they like and never put on weight?
- If you answered yes to any, or all, of the above questions, then what is contained within the pages No Diet Weight Loss will solve all your problems. This is a radical new way of achieving your perfect body weight and maintaining that weight PERMANENTLY - without diets, pills, potions or excessive exercise.

Dr Tom Smith said about this book:-

'This book is full of common sense and good advice on how to change one's life permanently to overcome all the habits that produce obesity. I will certainly recommend it to my patients. It gives people an excellent insight into themselves and how they have become overweight. It gives rational and sound advice on how to change their attitudes and lifestyle, not just so that they can be thinner, but happier with themselves, too. And it does this in a style that is easy to read, with humour and sympathy. An excellent book for everyone involved in obesity - and nowadays that means more than half of the adult population. I wish I had written it myself.'

ISBN 1-903784-10-7

88pp + CD